The Tao of Nutrition

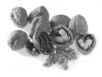

Other Books by Dr. Maoshing Ni

*Second Spring: Dr. Mao's Hundreds of Natural Secrets
for Women to Revitalize and Regenerate at Any Age*

*Secrets of Self-Healing: Harness Nature's Power to Heal
Common Ailments, Boost Your Vitality, and Achieve Optimum Wellness*

Secrets of Longevity: 101 Ways to Live to Be One Hundred

*Dr. Mao's Harmony Tai Chi:
Simple Practice for Health and Well-Being*

Chinese Herbology Made Easy

The Yellow Emperor's Classic of Medicine
(Editor and Translator)

Other Books by Cathy McNease

101 Vegetarian Delights (with Lily Chuang)

www.taostar.com
www.taoofwellness.com

THE TAO OF
NUTRITION

THIRD EDITION

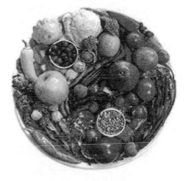

Maoshing Ni, Ph.D., O.M.D.
and Cathy McNease, B.S., Dipl. C.H.

Foreword by Hua-Ching Ni

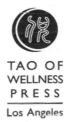

**TAO OF
WELLNESS
PRESS**

Los Angeles

Published by:
Tao of Wellness Press
An Imprint of SevenStar Communications
13315 W. Washington Boulevard , Suite 200
Los Angeles, CA 90066
www.taoofwellness.com

First Printing: January 1987
Second Printing: February 1989
Third Printing: June 1991
Fourth Printing: June 1993
Fifth Printing: March 1996
Sixth Printing: February 1998
Seventh Printing: June 2000
Eighth Printing: December 2004
Ninth Printing: April 2009
Tenth Printing April 2021

Publisher's Cataloging-in-Publication Data

Ni, Maoshing.

The Tao of nutrition / Maoshing Ni and Cathy McNease ; foreword by Hua-Ching Ni. — 3rd ed. — Los Angeles : Tao of Wellness Press, © 2009.

p. ; cm.

ISBN: 9781887575256
Includes bibliographical references and index.

1. Nutrition. 2. Health-Religious aspects—Taoism. 3. Diet therapy. I. McNease, Cathy. II. Title.

RA784 .N5 2008   2008921765
613.2—dc22   0806

Cover Design: Justina Krakowski Design
Interior Design & Production: Judith Liggett

Dedication

Eat not for the pleasure thou mayest find therein. Eat to increase thy strength. Eat to preserve the life thou has received from heaven.

Confucius

Acknowledgment

I would like to express my deepest gratitude to my father who has endowed me with the great tradition and knowledge of Chinese Nutrition so that I may be able to share it with everyone. A special appreciation is extended to master herbalist Cathy McNease who untiringly transcribed lectures, arranged and edited text, and provided important new additions to this third, expanded edition of *The Tao of Nutrition*.

We would also like to thank all our students, patients and friends for their valuable suggestions and feedback with the remedies in this book. To everyone who continues to support and promote natural medicine in the world, we are most grateful to all of you.

Disclaimer

This book is intended to inform the reader about the energetic and healing aspects of foods. It is the authors' earnest desire to further educate those who are open-minded about natural alternatives to healing. However, the remedies offered in this book are to be used at the reader's own discretion. If you wish to try the therapeutic approaches outlined in this book for a serious condition, it is best to first find a doctor of Chinese Medicine who can supervise your treatment.

About the Authors

Maoshing Ni is a doctor of Traditional Chinese Medicine, a bestselling author and an authority in Anti-Aging Medicine. Dr. Mao, as he is known to his patients and students, practices acupuncture and Chinese medicine with his brother, Dr. Daoshing Ni, and a team of associates at the Tao of Wellness in Santa Monica, California. He is cofounder and chancellor of Yo San University in Los Angeles, where he teaches the art and science of Wellness Medicine. Dr. Mao lectures internationally and has been featured on radio and television as well as on the pages of *The New York Times, Los Angeles Times*, and many other publications. He is the author of twelve books including *Secrets of Self Healing, Second Spring: Dr. Mao's Hundreds of Natural Secrets for Women to Revitalize and Regenerate at Any Age* and the bestselling *Secrets of Longevity*. For more information on his other publications, please visit www.taostar.com.

Cathy McNease holds a Diplomate in Chinese Herbology from the National Certification Commission for Acupuncture and Oriental Medicine (NCCAOM), a B.S. in Biology and Psychology from Western Michigan University and Master Herbalist certificates from Emerson College of Herbology in Canada and East-West Course of Herbology in Santa Cruz. She has co-authored two books and a distance learning course, *Traditional Chinese Nutrition*. She is currently on the faculties of Yo San University and Emperor's College of Traditional Oriental Medicine. In addition to her teaching profession she maintains a Chinese herbal pharmacy business, Best Blends Herbs.

Table of Contents

Foreword

THE KNOWLEDGE OF NUTRITION in China has roots that go back at least 6,000 years and is based on the principles of balance and harmony, as well as direct knowledge of the nature of individual foods. This knowledge was first gathered by spiritually achieved men and women who, by their own experiences, learned not only what properties specific foods contained, but also how to utilize them for the purposes of nutrition and longevity. Anyone who learns and uses this ancient, time-tested knowledge will find their health and longevity greatly enhanced.

Fu Shi, one of the great sages of ancient China, discovered eight categories of universal energy, which later came to be known as the *Ba Gua* or *Eight Trigrams*; this is a further division of the two main categories of natural energy known as Yin and Yang. The universe itself is an integration of these two interacting, mutually assisting and also somewhat opposing forces that are often expressed by the Tai Chi symbol.

The deepest reality of universal life is the inner meaning of Yin and Yang, and like Yin and Yang, the nature of the universe also tends to be both harmonious and balanced. Even events that could be conceptually classified as negative or conflicting, are only stages in the accomplishment of further harmonization. This is the truth expressed in the Tai Chi diagram.

Harmony and balance therefore, the principles of universal existence, became the foundation of cultural development in ancient China and were widely applied in public and private life as well as in spiritual practice. Many generations later, whatever expressed these natural universal qualities of balance, harmony and symmetry came to be known as Taoism; Tao being the way or path of universal harmony through integration.

Shen Nung, another wise leader who lived some time after Fu Shi, used these principles to develop herbal medicine and essential nutrition. After him came the Yellow Emperor, one of the greatest leaders in human history, who is considered the founder of Taoism. He further developed the contributions of the early sages, utilizing them in political as well as general life, especially in the realms of medicine and nutrition, and benefiting his hundred-year reign greatly by the guidance of this special knowledge.

Fu Shi, Shen Nung and the Yellow Emperor are great symbols of natural culture. Another symbolic figure of longevity is popular even now in Chinese culture. He is called Pung Tzu and is considered the founder of the art of Chinese cooking and nutrition. Pung Tzu learned all the arts of long life, including Dao-In, energy conducting exercises, and Fang Zhong, the art and discipline of sexual practices. Legend has it that Pung Tzu lived to be 800 years old and was still active in the reign of the Emperor Jou, around 1123 B.C.

As the spiritual descendents of these men of spiritual development and dedication to human development, we can still benefit today from their great achievements and contributions, as many have done before us. Through the traditional Chinese healing arts and herbal medicine, I myself have offered much useful knowledge and help to many people around the world. Although I taught a class on diet and nutrition several years ago, there was still a secret wish in my mind to do more in this area. Because of my busy schedule, I have not had time to do so, but fortunately my son Maoshing, had the same interest. Thus he has brought this book into your hands to fill the gap in my own work. It can be an important and useful tool in your life that will serve your health and spiritual development. With its support, I wish that each of you may become stronger every day.

Thank you,

Hua-Ching Ni

Preface

IN OUR RAPIDLY CHANGING SOCIETY, humans have lost their instinctive nature regarding healthy eating. People have a poor concept of what makes up a good diet. They thrive and rely on their taste buds and visual sensations for sustenance. In most cases they do not eat to live but rather live to eat.

Even more sadly, caught in their daily lives, many people make work, pleasure and sex a priority over what they eat. At the same time, mind-boggling numbers of fads and controversial dietary regimes add more confusion to their already uncertain dietary habits.

The Tao of Nutrition presents the wisdom of the ancient Chinese. Ancient people were much more aware of the environment and how their bodies reacted to their surroundings. They lived by the principle of being in harmony with nature and emphasized balance in every aspect of life, especially diet, the Yin and Yang of foods, and nourishment of the body. Their knowledge and experiences were passed down through generations and was further refined and systematized into what we today call Chinese nutrition.

Chinese nutrition is a healing system of its own. Not only is it a healing system, but it is also a disease-prevention system. The advantage of Chinese nutrition lies in its flexibility in adapting to every individual's needs, and treating the whole person rather than just the symptoms.

Chinese nutrition differs from modern Western nutrition in that it does not rely on analyzing the chemical constituents of each food; rather it determines the properties or energies of each food and combination. It takes into consideration the season, method of preparation, geographical location, and information that is in accord with the natural principles of life and balance.

It is hoped that the readers of this book will gain understanding of their bodies, their surroundings, and their diet. So here it is, the essence of the art and science of Chinese nutrition. With this book in your hands, you can acquire insight and be the master of your own body. Start now to achieve and maintain health, vitality, and longevity.

How To Use This Book

THIS BOOK CONTAINS five sections: The first section deals with the theories and philosophies of Chinese nutrition. Section Two describes over 130 common foods in detail–their energetic properties, their therapeutic actions, and individual remedies. Section Three is a remedial section that gives recommendations for various medical conditions. Sections Four and Five contain recipes and meal plans.

It is strongly recommended that readers familiarize themselves thoroughly with the first section in order to understand the basic philosophies of Chinese nutrition. With that understanding, one is able to more efficiently utilize the specific knowledge given in the remaining sections.

Another way readers may find this book useful is to refer to conditions that apply to them. They may either choose to look up a condition in Section Three and follow the recommendations given there or check the index for listings of the condition.

For example, if you look up *Headache* in Section Three, you will find the following therapeutic remedies to choose from:

For headaches due to common cold or flu:

1. Make tea from ginger and green onions, boiling for 5 minutes. Drink and allow body to sweat.

2. Steam aching portion of head over mint and cinnamon tea that is boiling. Dry head afterwards, avoiding drafts.

3. Make tea from chrysanthemum flowers and cassia seeds and drink.

4. Mash buckwheat meal into a paste and apply to painful area until it sweats.

5. Drink green tea.

6. Make rice porridge and add garlic and green onions. Eat while hot, and then get under blankets and sweat.

For headaches due to high blood pressure, menstrual cycles, emotional stress or tension, or migraines:

1. Make carrot juice. If headache is on the left side, squirt carrot juice into left nostril; if on the right side, squirt into right nostril; if both sides are painful, squirt into both nostrils.

2. Take lemon juice and ½ T. baking soda mixed in a glass of water and drink.

3. Make tea of Chinese prunes, mint, and green tea.

4. Make tea of oyster shells and chrysanthemum flowers, slowly boiling the shells for 1 ½ hours, then adding the flowers for the last 30 minutes.

5. Mash peach kernels and walnuts. Mix with rice wine and lightly roast; take 2 T. three times daily.

6. Rinse head with warm water, gradually increasing the temperature to hot.

After studying the entire book, one will gain an insight into maintaining balance and harmony between one's body and the environment and ultimately will achieve health, happiness and longevity.

Section One

Introduction to Chinese Nutrition

Energetic Properties

Chinese nutrition applies the traditional healing properties of foods to correct disharmonies within the body. Over the course of several millennia, countless experiences were gathered using food for prevention and healing of disease. This treasure was passed along as an important healing art, within the body of information known as Traditional Chinese Medicine.

Chinese nutrition differs from Western nutrition in that it does not talk about the biochemical nature of food. Rather, Chinese nutrition deals on an energetic level where **balance is the key**. Foods are selected according to their energetic qualities such as warming, cooling, drying, or lubricating. Thus, Chinese nutrition would seek to warm the coldness, cool the heat, dry the dampness, lubricate the dryness, and so forth.

By carefully studying the individual's imbalances, one would choose the appropriate foods to bring about a balanced state of health. For example, for an excessive individual who is exhibiting conditions of heat in the body, cooling foods would be appropriate. For a deficient individual who tends toward coldness, warming foods would be chosen. In this way, balance is achieved.

Foods all have specific inherent qualities determined by the effect the food has on the body. Then the method of preparation further enhances or neutralizes the foods. Generally speaking, warming foods raise metabolism and cooling foods lower metabolism. Balance in the diet is essential for good health.

Yin and Yang

It is a universal law that everything is constantly changing, except for the fundamental governing laws of life. This principle applies to the universe surrounding us as well as the inner universe of our bodies. The ancient Chinese developed ways of looking at these changes to better understand them. One such theory is that everything in the universe consists of two opposite yet complementary aspects. This is called the *Theory of Yin and Yang*. Yin and Yang exist relative to one another and are also in a state of change at any given time; they are not static conditions. Day and night is a good example of this. When Yin and Yang are out of balance, diseases or disharmonies occur.

Within the body, Yin and Yang are often referred to as the body's water and fire. These descriptions are very useful in determining the relative nature of both the individual and the energies of foods. The application of Chinese nutrition necessitates determining the body type of the individual. He or she may be the *cold type*, considered of a Yin nature, the *hot type*, considered Yang, or commonly a mixture. Some significant questions to determine this may be as follows, with the Yang tendencies listed first: *male or female? feel hot or cold? drawn to hot or cold foods? thirst or no thirst? constipated or loose stools? dark or pale urine? red or pale face and tongue?*

We are all a mixture of Yin and Yang, although we may be predominantly one or the other. Thus, Yang persons need relatively more Yin, or cooling foods whereas, Yin types need relatively more Yang, or warming foods. Chinese nutrition categorizes foods according to the observed reactions within the body. Easily observable changes occur according to the warming or cooling nature of a food. Foods are categorized as Hot, Warm, Neutral, Cool or Cold. (See *Chart 1: Energetic Properties of Foods,* pgs. 215-218.)

Typical symptoms of the *hot type* or *Yang type* person could include the following: red complexion, easy to sweat, always hot, dominating, aggressive or outgoing personality, coarseness, loud voice, dry mouth, thirst, affinity to cold liquids, ferocious appetite, constipation, foul breath, scanty and dark urine, sometimes dry cough with thick yellow sputum, easily angered, very emotional, irritability, insomnia, and in women, early and heavy menstruation with bright red blood.

Typical symptoms of the *cold type* or *Yin type* person could include the following: paleness, coldness, disdains cold liquids, likes warm liquids, low energy, loose stools, sleeps a lot, feeble and weak voice, introverted personality, white and copious sputum, lack of appetite, copious and clear urine, dizziness, and edema.

To bring about balance and counteract the symptoms, *hot type* persons would use primarily cooling foods such as wheat, mung beans, watermelon, fresh fruit juices, and many of the vegetables. *Cold type* persons would achieve balance by regularly including the warming foods in their diet, such as garlic, ginger, onions, black beans, lamb and chicken. Accordingly, *hot types* would avoid hot, spicy foods, while *cold types* would avoid cold, raw foods.

Yin and Yang also apply to the organs of our bodies. Those which are considered solid, or with substance, are considered Yin. These include Heart, Spleen, Liver, Lungs, and Kidneys. Those which are considered hollow, active in transportation, are considered Yang. These include Large and Small Intestines, Gall Bladder, Stomach, and Urinary Bladder. Further descriptions of each organ and their energetic components will follow. (See *Chart 2: Five Elements Correspondences*, pg. 219-220.)

Your Body Is The Greatest Healer

Many people are overfed and undernourished. We are constantly bombarded by information on nutrition from food companies, current faddists, and diet cultists, yet the picture is very incomplete. According to the Chinese point of view, the body is looked at as a whole, working together in harmony.

Just as every screw and bolt on a machine has an important purpose, if one part is broken the whole suffers. Our body is a very intricate machine that works together as a whole.

Western medicine tends to focus on symptoms and the diseased part of the body. It tries to attack and kill the diseased cells, not taking into account *how* those cells became diseased. It is not just because the cells are exposed to viruses and bacteria. We are constantly being exposed; even our mouths are full of bacteria. Yet why is it that some people break down and get sick and others do not when both are exposed to the same pathogens?

Our body is equipped with a healing mechanism that is greater than any invention. It is unique in that it has a system that can repair the body's disharmonies, given the opportunity to do so. Through inappropriate lifestyle, diet, thoughts, and actions, we abuse the workings of this delicate system. Always keep in mind that the body's own healing system is very powerful. Suppressing a headache with aspirin does not take away the underlying cause. The headache is a warning of some disharmony. Thus, we should work on the underlying cause and use natural healing methods to enhance the immune system so the body can heal itself.

The focus of Traditional Chinese Medicine is to help the body to heal, not interfere with the healing process. Often our surroundings do not give us the proper chance to heal ourselves because we are bombarded with chemicals in our soil, food, water, and urban environment. These chemicals can accumulate in the liver and become very toxic.

Significant chemical pollution occurs in meats. Meat animals are routinely injected with steroids such as bovine growth hormone to fatten them quickly and made them produce more milk. Antibiotics, including penicillin and sulfa, are used to control rampant diseases. These drug residues remain in meat and milk and cause health problems for the consumer. Hormones can cause men to become more feminine and have problems with impotency and sterility and women to experience premature aging and general disharmonies in their endocrine systems and menstrual cycles.

Traditional Chinese View of the Body

According to Traditional Chinese Medicine (TCM), the human as an intricate whole is made up of the following essential components: Chi, or vital energy, blood, body fluids; Jing, or the essence of life; and Shen, or spirit. If any one of these components is missing, you cannot have life.

Chi comes in many forms with many different actions. In general, Chi is like life force. The body is a network of Chi pathways called meridians. In a healthy person, Chi or energy flows evenly along these channels. When the energy becomes blocked, disease results. Acupuncture can be of great value in facilitating the flow of energy through these pathways. Chi, the Yang component, is closely related to blood, the Yin component. Blood supplies nutrition to the body and nourishes Chi. Movement of blood is dependent upon Chi.

Body fluids are of two types: Jin are the thin, refined fluids such as sweat, tears, and tissue fluids and Ye are the thick, lubricating fluids such as spinal fluid and synovial, or joint fluids.

Jing is the essence of life found in the egg, sperm, marrow, and brain (the sea of marrow) and is stored in the Kidneys. At the time of conception, the fetus absorbs this vital essence from the egg and the sperm. All of our chromosomes at that time give us our Jing. Thus, we are born with a certain amount. Throughout our lives we use up our Jing until we die. Our fast-paced lifestyle uses up Jing at a very rapid rate. For this reason women can have problems with menstruation, go through an earlier menopause and cannot safely bear children for as many years as in more natural cultures.

Spiritual cultivation is very important for the proper development and preservation of our Jing, which is stored in the Kidneys. The Shen, or spirit, gives us intuition, instincts, and the ability to comprehend. Shen is housed in the Heart.

Organs of the Body

TCM views the body organs as couples consisting of a Yin organ and a Yang organ. Each pair also has energetic correlations that we may not necessarily associate with the physical organ. For example, the Kidneys in Chinese medicine would also include functions of the reproductive organs. Each pair of organs is associated with one of the five energies called the Five Elements: Wood, Fire, Earth, Metal, and Water. (See *Chart 2*, pgs. 219-220.) The quality of the element is reflected in its organ pair.

The pair related to the Wood element is the Liver and Gall Bladder. The Liver houses the soul, controls tendons, stores blood, manifests externally in the eyes, and is responsible for keeping energy flowing. Thus, when the energy is obstructed, look to the Liver. Anger, frustration, and depression relates to the Liver. The Gall Bladder stores and excretes bile, protects the nervous system from overreaction, and helps to normalize a person emotionally. Gall Bladder weakness may manifest as difficulty making decisions.

Corresponding to the Fire element are the Heart and Small Intestines. The Heart houses the Shen, governs blood, has taste as its sensory function, externally manifests in the tongue, and joy (mania) is its related emotion. The Small Intestines absorb fluids. As one of the hollow organs, they are responsible for the transporting of excretion.

Also related to the Fire element are the Triple Heater, or Sanjiao, and the Pericardium. These are functions rather than organs. The Triple Heater is responsible for communication between the three cavities in the trunk and helps with fluid metabolism in the body. The Pericardium surrounds and protects the Heart.

Corresponding to the element of Earth is the Spleen and Stomach pair. The Spleen transforms and transports food into usable food essence (the waste is transported to the intestines), produces blood, opens to the mouth, and controls muscles. It is also responsible for keeping blood in the vessels. Thus, bruising easily is a sign of weak Spleen function. The related emotion is worry, or excessive thinking. Reference made to the Spleen in the Chinese system also includes functions of the pancreas. The Stomach breaks down and *ripens* the food and then transports it downward.

The pair corresponding to the Metal element is the Lungs and Large Intestines. The main functions of the Lungs are breathing, regulating water metabolism, and descending and dispersing Chi throughout the body. The Lungs open out to the nose and control the skin, pores, and hair on the skin. Sadness is the related emotion. The Large Intestines excrete wastes from the body and absorb water.

Related to the Water element are the Kidneys and Urinary Bladder. The Kidneys store Jing, are responsible for growth, development, and reproduction. The Kidneys also produce marrow, form the brain and spinal cord, control bones, open to the ears, and balance body fluid metabolism. The related emotion is fear. The Urinary Bladder stores and excretes urine.

Five Elements

A basic theory in the Chinese view of the universe is the Five Elements Theory, or the Five Energy Transformations. (See *Chart 3: Five Energetic Transformations*, p. 221.) This view gives us a helpful framework for understanding the ever-changing world, the inner relationships of change, and the interconnectedness of all things. The five elements, Wood, Fire, Earth, Metal, and Water, connect in that sequence for what is called the *creation cycle*. This cycle occurs in nature as well as within our bodies. In nature, rub two pieces of wood together and create fire; fire burns to ash and becomes earth; from earth we dig up metal; melt the metal to liquid and make water; put a seed into the water and it germinates a tree and creates wood. The cycle is circular.

In the creation cycle, the creator element is the mother who gives birth to the son element. Thus, if the son is weak or deficient, we can tonify or nourish the mother and thereby benefit the son. If there is not enough Fire (corresponding to the Heart), we would strengthen the Wood organ (the Liver) with the proper foods or herbs.

In ancient times, these correspondences were made by observing that nature and our bodies work similarly. In nature the Five Elements can be correlated to the seasons as follows: Wood corresponds to spring; Fire corresponds to summer; Earth corresponds to late summer and the time between seasons; Metal corresponds to autumn; and Water corresponds to winter.

There is a useful relationship between food colors and the elements and corresponding body systems. White foods nourish the Lungs; black and dark blue foods nourish the Kidneys; green foods nourish the Liver; yellow and orange foods nourish the Spleen and Stomach; red foods nourish the Heart. Thus, a person with weak digestion, a Spleen weakness, should include plenty of the yellow and orange foods such as sweet potatoes and winter squashes, as these are the colors that correspond to the Earth element. Someone with Heart weakness would do well to eat more red foods such as tomatoes and hawthorn berries, as red corresponds to the Fire element.

Another relationship that occurs within the Five Elements is the *control cycle*. (See *Chart 3*, pg. 221). It goes like this: we take wood, for example a tree, whose roots grow into the earth; we take earth and build a dam to control water; water puts out the fire; fire melts down the metal; metal makes the ax that cuts the wood. If the Wood element (Liver) becomes excessive and manifests as hypertension, red eyes and a headache, we may want to strengthen or tonify the Metal element (Lungs) to control the Wood.

The creation and control cycles occur as natural phenomenon, keeping life in balance. However, when any one of the elements is either too strong or too weak, disharmony results. Keep in mind as you use the Five Elements Theory that there are always exceptions to the rule.

The Five Tastes

The physical sensation of taste has its significance in Chinese medicine. Taste is classified into five flavors, although in the text below you will actually find seven. These five tastes are: sour, sweet, bitter, pungent, and salty. The other two are bland, which falls under the sweet category, and astringent, which falls under the sour category.

When a substance such as a food or an herb goes into the gastrointestinal tract to be digested, the sour taste is said to be absorbed by the Liver and Gall Bladder, the bitter taste by the Heart and Small Intestines, the sweet taste by the Spleen and Stomach, the pungent taste by the Lungs and Large Intestines, and the salty taste by the Kidneys and Urinary Bladder. Therefore, foods and herbs with different energies and tastes are assimilated into the body to nourish different organs.

Take the example of someone with digestive difficulties as in a weakness of Spleen and Stomach. He or she often likes to eat sweets. Contrary to Western medicine, in which those with digestive weakness are advised against sweets intake, Chinese medicine utilizes foods, such as yam or winter squash, that are actually slightly sweet and strengthen the weakness of Spleen and Stomach. Thus, consumption of foods with various tastes will benefit those organs that correspond to these tastes.

• **Pungent** is a taste that has functions of dispersing, invigorating, and promoting circulation. Its function of dispersing is mainly used to disperse pathogens from the exterior of the body, such as we see in common colds and flu. Its function of invigorating is to promote circulation of Chi, blood and body fluids. In Chinese medicine, disease is the result of stagnation; therefore, foods that have this pungent taste will promote and invigorate circulation of Chi, blood and body fluids. The pathological condition of stagnation can be seen as local pain, irregular and/or painful menstruation, edema, tumors, and so on. The pungent taste, because of its dispersing quality also acts to open the pores and promote sweating. This is a way to expel the pathogen from the body. Examples of pungent tasting foods are ginger, garlic and mint.

• **Sour** taste has absorbing, consolidating, and astringent functions. It functions in stopping abnormal discharge of body fluids and substances as in the condition of excessive perspiration, diarrhea, seminal emission, spermatorrhea, and enuresis. Examples of sour foods are Chinese sour plum, lemon and vinegar.

• **Astringent** taste falls under the sour taste category and its actions are very similar to that of the sour taste.

• **Bitter** substances have the action of drying dampness and dispersing obstructions. Often bitter also clears heat, so bitter aids conditions like dampness and edema. Its function of dispersing obstruction can be utilized for a cough due to Chi stagnation and so forth. Examples of bitter-tasting foods are rhubarb, apricot kernels, and kale.

• **Salty** taste has the function of softening and dissolving hardenings. It also moistens and lubricates the intestines. Body symptoms such as lumps, nodes, masses, and cysts can be softened and dissolved by salty substances. An example can be seen in goiter, which is treated by seaweed, a representative of salty food. Also, in cases of constipation, one can drink salt water to lubricate the intestines and promote evacuation.

• **Sweet** taste has the action of tonifying, harmonizing and decelerating. In cases of fatigue or deficiency, sweet substances have a reinforcing and strengthening action. Deficiencies may occur in different aspects of the body, such as insufficiency of Chi, blood, Yin or Yang. Specific organs may suffer from weakness as well. This is why one is drawn to sweets when he or she is experiencing low energy. Sweet taste is also used to decelerate, which means to relax. It is used in conditions of acute pain to help relax and hence, ease the pain. Sweet foods and herbs can harmonize as an antidote or counterbalance undesirable effects from some herbs. Examples of sweet-tasting foods are yams, corn and rice.

• **Bland** taste falls under the sweet taste category. It tends to be diuretic, promotes urination and relieves edema. An example of a bland-tasting food is pearl barley.

The Eight Differentiations

In order to more clearly understand the energy of the patient and the nature and location of the disease, the Chinese have developed the Eight Differentiations system of diagnosis. *Internal* and *external* serves to locate the area of disease. *Deficiency* and *excess* determine the relative strength of the patient or the disease. *Cold* and *hot* give indications of the nature of the individual and/or the pathogens. *Yin* and *Yang* give the overall picture of the condition. Together these eight differentiations can provide an accurate picture of both the individual being treated and the disease at hand. A mixture of symptoms can be confusing. The Eight Differentiations provide a basis for understanding seeming contradictions in the symptoms. A practitioner of Traditional Chinese Medicine would make an evaluation based on the tongue and pulse readings and the presenting signs and symptoms.

Causes of Disease

In Traditional Chinese Medicine, the cause of disease is said to be of an *external* or *internal* source. Just below the surface of the skin lies a layer of energy that acts as a protective shield. In a healthy person this shield is strong and without gaps as a barrier of protection should be. It is impervious to external factors. If, however, there are weak spots in this shield and external factors can penetrate into the body, we have disease. This shield is part of the immune system. If one's immune system is strong, one does not catch the pathogen. For example, some people have the AIDS virus and show no symptoms of it; others catch it and soon die. That is the difference between strong Chi and weak Chi.

In the Chinese perception of disease, external causes of diseases include the following environmental conditions: cold, heat, summer heat, dryness, dampness, and wind. In Western thinking, we would put viruses and bacteria in this category.

Diseases can also arise as a result of internal factors. These include the emotions: joy (mania), grief, anger, depression, worry, melancholy, and fear. These reflect the mental state induced by one's environment. That in itself does not cause disease. However, when emotions are very intense or long lasting, disharmony or disease can result. Mental attitude is very important for good health. By calming one's mind, many physical problems disappear.

An interesting survey done in China on a group of cancer patients showed that 95% had been physically or mentally tortured during the Cultural Revolution (1965-1975). During that harsh period, intellectuals were tortured; even husbands and wives betrayed each other for the sake of the Communist Party. You could not trust anyone with your innermost feelings and thoughts. These people built up frustration, depression, and anger, and these destructive emotions in turn became cancer. Isolation and inability to express emotions is very destructive to one's health.

It is important to recognize the role of emotional balance in maintaining good health. We must have a channel to release excessive emotions, be it exercises such as tai chi chuan or chi gong, breathing techniques, acupuncture, meditation, or walking. These activities can help to regulate emotions and promote more inner peace.

Other causes of disease include traumatic injury, stagnant blood or mucus, improper exercise, improper activities, and improper diet. Traumatic injuries include accidents, incisions, sprains, burns, and animal or insect bites. Stagnancy of the blood and mucus cause blocks in the energy pathways; a good example is tumors.

Either too much or too little exercise can cause disease. Improper activities include excessive sex, overworking, and overexertion. Excessive sex is particularly injurious to the Kidneys, the store-house of our Jing. Improper diet can be eating too little for proper nourishment of the body, overeating, or eating too much of the wrong foods, such as too much raw, cold, greasy, or spicy foods.

Overeating is a very common imbalance and can cause many diseases. We frequently overeat because we do not know how to eat and tend to eat very fast. By chewing food slowly and properly, the body will naturally tell us when to stop. People also reach out to food and use it as an escape. Eating in a relaxed frame of mind is essential to good digestion and assimilation of nutrients.

It has been found in animal experiments that if one group is allowed to eat as much as desired and another group is starved every second day, the first group had five times more tendency toward spontaneous cancer. Statistically, the United States leads the world in both protein consumption per person and the incidence of cancer. Protein is needed, but an excessive amount causes problems. An over consumption of meat protein will also result in a high percentage of fat in the diet, another significant contributor to disease. Meat companies have led us to believe that we need far more protein than is really healthy. Moderation is essential to good health.

A study conducted from 1983-1988 of 6,500 people from 65 regions across China, showed the impact that regular exercise and a low-fat, high-fiber diet have on maintaining good health. This was the largest study of its kind to date. The findings of the China Project on Nutrition, Health, and the Environment were published in 1990 as *Diet, Lifestyle, and Morality in China*. This project was under the direction of T. Colin Campbell of Cornell University, in collaboration with researchers from Oxford University, Chinese Academy of Preventive Medicine, and Chinese Academy of Medical Sciences, both in Beijing.

The results suggested that the healthiest diet would contain a minimum of 80-90% plant foods. Those in the Chinese countryside, who get only about 10-15% of their calories and 7% of their total protein from animal products, had low incidence of heart disease, colon cancer, and osteoporosis. The study showed that when the rural dweller moved to the city and adopted the city lifestyle and higher fat diet (30%), diseases increased.

The Western approach to diseases is to kill bacteria and suppress the symptoms, thus driving the disease deeper into the body. The Chinese way supports the body and lets it do the killing of the pathogen. Supporting the body with tonification reinforces the body's healing energy. The body can heal itself if given the chance although we may need to give it assistance through proper nutrition or herbal medicine.

Fasting or light eating is sometimes recommended during an illness, such as a cold, so digestion of heavy foods will not detract from the body's healing process. In many traditions throughout the world, a thin, soupy grain porridge, or *congee*, is given during illness. This is very easy to digest, and thus the body can draw on its resources to heal. The antibiotic route, on the other hand, weakens the immune system, makes one prone to illness, causes the immune system to become lazy, and generally interferes with the natural healing process.

There are many supportive measures that can be taken with food and herbs. In many instances, we need to support the body while concurrently detoxifying or sedating it. This is the Chinese approach to disease. For cancer patients in some hospitals in China, doctors combine the killing aspects of chemotherapy and radiation with the supportive measures of Traditional Chinese Medicine, including proper diet, herbs, chi gong exercises and acupuncture. This has produced a longer life expectancy than the conventional killing approach alone. Some hospitals treat cancer patients solely with Chinese medicine; this group often shows the longest life expectancy including many total remissions.

Prevention of Disease

As we increase our awareness of health, we can maintain a state of balance within the body, and become more responsible for our health. Too often we suffer from our inappropriate actions and thoughts. Chinese nutrition stresses prevention of disease. Written 2,000-3,000 years ago, *The Yellow Emperor's Classic of Internal Medicine* says, "A doctor who treats a disease after it has happened is a mediocre doctor. But a doctor who treats a disease before it happens is a superior doctor." Doctors were considered to be teachers who taught their patients how to be healthy and spiritually upright. Success was measured by vibrant health. We as individuals choose to be one kind of doctor or the other.

Traditionally, herbs have been used to preserve good health and prevent disease. Many of the tonifying herbs are used for this purpose over a long period of time. The tonic herbs are further categorized into Yin, Yang, Blood and Chi tonics, and lend themselves well to preparations with foods, such as soups, stew and porridges. Incorporating the appropriate herbs into the diet on a regular basis can provide great benefit to health.

The use of herbs as food has a long history in China. The first Chinese Materia Medica, *Shen-Nong Herbal Classic,* categorizes herbs into three groups. The first group was called food herbs, which were eaten as a part of the diet for general nourishment, maintenance of health, and prevention of disease. Taoist hermits called these herbs immortal foods and described them as producing effects that rejuvenate health, prolong life, restore youth, and increase clarity. They often used them as the main part of their diet, along with some fruits, nuts and seeds. Later sections of this book describe some of these food herbs. For additional reading on food herbs and recipes, refer to the Bibliography at the end of this book.

The other two groups of herbs were called medicinal herbs, which were dispensed to patients in an individual formula based on each patient's constitution, environment and medical condition, by a traditional Chinese medical professional.

Prevention of disease includes proper nutrition, exercise, emotional balance, and nourishing our spirit. As we nourish body, mind, and spirit we maintain a state of balance. Preventative maintenance is the most sensible route to take. As The Yellow Emperor states,

> The sages of ancient times emphasized not the treatment of disease, but rather the prevention of its occurrence. To administer medicine to disease that has already developed and to suppress revolts that have already begun is comparable to the behavior of one who begins to dig a well after he has become thirsty or one who begins to forge weapons after he has engaged in battle. Would these actions not be too late?

Guidelines for a Balanced Diet

As every body is unique, there will always be variations according to individual needs. A few basic guidelines, however, are appropriate as we seek a way of eating that creates balance and harmony. Frame of mind is of utmost importance at mealtime; relax and slowly chew your food for optimal digestion and assimilation. The dinner table is not the place to discuss the day's problems. Chewing is a major part of digestion. Remember, your stomach does not have teeth. Digestion, particularly of the starches, begins in the mouth. Foods that are difficult to thoroughly chew, such as sesame seeds, should be ground before eating. Fruits digest quickly, while meats and other proteins take more time to digest.

The preferred ways of preparing foods are steaming, stir-frying in water, stewing (boiling, as in soups), or baking. Steaming leaves the food in its most natural state, while baking creates more heat and would be the best method for cold conditions. Even the best quality oils become difficult to digest when heated. So, if oil is desired, put it on after the food is cooked.

Foods should be eaten in their wholeness, when possible. Only peel fruits or vegetables if the peel is hard to digest or contaminated with chemical sprays. Search out organically grown foods to avoid the toxic chemical residues of commercial growing processes. To clean foods thoroughly, one may wash them in salt water. Also avoid irradiated or microwaved foods, if possible. The best utensils for cooking in are glass, earthenware, or stainless steel. One should avoid cooking in aluminum or copper; these metals can easily leach into the food.

The food one eats should follow the seasons and should be grown locally. Nature has the perfect plan for providing the appropriate foods in each given season. The fruits and vegetables that ripen in the summertime tend to be on the cooling side. In wintertime we will tend toward a more warming diet. Also, one should eat a wide variety of foods for good balance.

Most vegetables should be at least lightly cooked because raw vegetables tend to be difficult to digest. Foods should never be eaten cold because cold foods *put out the digestive fire*, so to speak. This is particularly upsetting to the female menstrual cycle as the stomach sits right beside the liver which is responsible for storing blood. Cooling off the stomach can lead to a stagnant blood condition and a difficult menstrual period. Frozen foods, such as ice cream and iced drinks, are very unhealthy. Neither should we consume foods that are so hot that they burn the mouth or stomach.

It is best to stop eating before becoming full. Also, eating just before retiring is not a good idea; one should eat the last meal at least three hours before going to bed. This will not only result in better digestion, but also a more restful sleep. Late eating also tends to be stored as unwanted pounds. One should wake up with a good appetite for breakfast. This is the meal that provides us with the fuel or energy for much of the day, so make breakfast a very nutritious meal.

Nuts and seeds contain a large proportion of oil and should be eaten as fresh as possible and kept refrigerated. Because most people do not chew nuts well, grinding them into powder makes them easier to digest.

Beans should be soaked prior to cooking for at least a few hours; always discard the soaking water and cook them in fresh water. Small beans like lentils and peas tend to be easier to digest than large beans like lima or kidney beans. For a person with particularly weak digestion, it is best to cook grains *soupy* with additional water and cooking time. You may use up to ten parts water per one part grain.

Always avoid highly processed foods and keep meals as simple as possible. A balanced diet would consist of the following on a regular basis:

Whole grains including rice, millet, barley, wheat, oats, corn, rye, quinoa, amaranth, etc. This group of foods will account for about 40% of the diet.

Freshly prepared vegetables including dark leafy greens, cabbage, broccoli, celery, root vegetables, etc. This group of foods will account for about 40% of the diet.

Fresh fruits will be consumed when in season but generally no more than 10% of the diet. Fruits can be a great snack or sweet treat.

Legumes/seeds/nuts including peas, beans, tofu, peanuts, lentils, sunflower seeds, almonds, walnuts, etc. This group will account for about 10-20% of the vegetarian diet and a lesser portion of the meat-inclusive diet.

Animal products include dairy foods, meat, fish, poultry, and eggs. They should be no more than 10% of the diet if one chooses to include them. Attempt to locate growers who do not use drugs or inhumane practices on the animals.

Seaweeds including nori, wakame, dulse, kombu, hiziki, and arame. This is a valuable mineral source, consumed in small amounts (a small handful dry), and of particular value to those vegetarians who refrain from eating dairy foods.

As strictly as possible, avoid consuming the following: chemical preservatives, additives, colorings and flavorings, MSG, fried or greasy foods, coffee, ice cream and excessive sugar.

The United States Department of Agriculture (USDA) has adopted a Food Pyramid that shows food proportions for a healthy diet. It is very similar to the food group proportions used in Chinese Nutrition. Grains, beans, vegetables and fruits constitute the base of the pyramid and majority of the diet, while meat and dairy foods, eaten in small proportions, are at the top. This shows people how to make changes in their dietary habits and ways of looking at food.

Section Two

Foods

Please note: In this section, food is frequently measured in grams.
Twenty-eight grams = one ounce

Vegetables

Alfalfa Sprouts
Nature/Taste: cool and slightly bitter

Actions: benefits Spleen and Stomach, dispels dampness, lubricates intestines

Conditions: swelling, constipation, skin lesions

Folk Remedies:
1. **Swelling** – boil tea and drink three times daily.
2. **Constipation** – eat raw alfalfa sprouts.
3. **Skin lesions** – apply mashed alfalfa sprouts; change poultice 3-4 times daily.

Artichoke
Nature/Taste: sweet, bitter, cooling

Actions: regulates Liver Chi, clears Liver heat, promotes digestion, benefits Liver and Gall Bladder, dries dampness

Conditions: headache, melancholy, high blood pressure, indigestion, bloating, gas, abdominal pain, high cholesterol, skin itch, dysbiosis, candidiasis, diarrhea

Folk Remedies:
1. **Headache** – make tea by boiling one whole artichoke with 1/2 cup fresh peppermint leaves in 4 cups water for 20 minutes. Make sure lid is tightly covered. Drink a cup every 3 hours until headache is relieved
2. **Yeast infection/candidiasis** – eat a steamed artichoke daily for 2 weeks
3. **High cholesterol** – make soup with diced artichoke hearts, sliced ginger and 1/2 head of cabbage. Eat a bowl daily.
4. **Liver problem/jaundice** – make tea by boiling 1/2 cup artichoke leaves in 4 cups water for 30 minutes. Strain and drink 1 cup of tea 3 times a day.

Asparagus

Nature/Taste: cool, sweet and bitter

Actions: clears heat, detoxifies, promotes blood circulation, clears lungs

Conditions: constipation, cancer, hypertension, high blood cholesterol, arteriosclerosis, bronchitis

Folk Remedies:

1. **High cholesterol, hypertension, and arteriosclerosis** – drink one glass daily of pureed asparagus juice, including the pulp; add one teaspoon of honey.
2. **Breast cancer** – boil asparagus with dandelions; drink the liquid and apply the solids to the area.
3. **Constipation** – eat asparagus with cabbage, lightly steamed.

Bamboo Shoots

Nature/Taste: cool and sweet

Actions: strengthens the stomach, relieves food retention, resolves mucus, promotes diuresis, cuts or emulsifies fats, relieves alcohol intoxication, eases thirst caused by measles

Conditions: diabetes, indigestion, stomach distention and fullness due to greasy foods, diarrhea, dysentery, rectal prolapse, edema

Contraindications: not to be used after giving birth as they may trigger the cleansing of an old illness, manifesting in skin lesions.

Folk Remedies:

1. **Diarrhea, dysentery, and rectal prolapse** – cook bamboo shoots with rice.
2. **Swelling due to kidney, heart, or liver disease** – drink tea of bamboo shoots and winter melon skin.
3. **Diabetes** – blend bamboo shoots and celery juice, warm up and drink one cup twice daily. Eat plenty of bamboo shoots.

4. **Stomach distension and fullness** – make tea from bamboo shoots, ginger and orange peel and drink.

Beets

Nature/Taste: cool and sweet

Actions: nourishes blood, tonifies the Heart, calms the spirit, lubricates the intestines, cleanses the liver

Conditions: anemia, heart weakness, irritability, restlessness, habitual constipation, herpes, liver intoxification from drugs or alcohol

Contraindications: not for someone with a history of kidney stones due to the oxalic acid content.

Folk Remedies:

1. **Constipation** – make beet soup, or combine beets with cabbage.
2. **Blood deficiency** – cook beets with black beans and peanuts.
3. **Liver cleansing** – drink beet top tea, or combine with dandelions and make tea.
4. **Herpes** – do a three-day fast with vegetable broth* and beet top tea.

* Basic vegetable broth for detoxification can be made by simmering carrots and carrot tops, celery, dandelions, asparagus, and squash.

Bell Pepper

Nature/Taste: slightly warm, pungent and sweet

Actions: strengthens stomach, improves appetite, promotes blood circulation, removes stagnant food, reduces swelling

Conditions: indigestion, decreased appetite, swelling, food retention, frostbite

Folk Remedies:

1. **Indigestion and food retention** – make green pepper tea.

2. **Frostbite** – wash affected area in bell pepper and cinnamon tea, and drink the tea.
3. **Decreased appetite and anorexia** – mix bell pepper with black pepper and dry fry (no oil). Or lightly fry chunks of bell pepper with oil.

Bok Choy

Nature/Taste: cool, pungent and sweet

Actions: clears heat, lubricates the intestines, removes stagnant food, quenches thirst, promotes digestion

Conditions: food retention, constipation, indigestion, diabetes

Folk Remedies:
1. **Food retention** – boil tea or soup from bok choy and orange peel.
2. **Indigestion** – eat pickled bok choy.
3. **Constipation** – cook bok choy with beets.
4. **Thirst** – drink bok choy and cucumber juice.

Broccoli

Nature/Taste: cool and sweet

Actions: clears heat, promotes diuresis, brightens eyes, clears summer heat problems. This vegetable is weak in action.

Conditions: conjunctivitis, nearsightedness, difficult urination, irritability

Folk Remedies:
1. **Clear heat** – eat lightly steamed broccoli.
2. **Conjunctivitis (pink eye)** – drink carrot and broccoli tea.
3. **Urinary difficulty** – combine broccoli with Chinese cabbage and make soup.

Burdock Root (Gobo)

Nature/Taste: cool, pungent and bitter

Actions: clears heat, dispels wind, brightens vision

Conditions: common cold of the wind-heat type, sore throat, measles, conjunctivitis, mumps

Contraindications: not to be used in cases of diarrhea.

Folk Remedies:

1. **Conjunctivitis (pink eye)** – boil tea and expose eyes to the steam, then drink the tea.
2. **Common cold and measles** – drink burdock tea and sweat.
3. **Mumps** – make burdock and dandelion tea, apply locally and drink the tea.

Cabbage, Red or Green

Nature/Taste: cool and sweet

Actions: clears heat, lubricates intestines, stops cough

Conditions: constipation, whooping cough, hot flashes, common colds, frostbite

Folk Remedies:

1. **Common cold** – combine ¼ head cabbage and three green onions, boil 10 minutes and drink the liquid, and sweat.
2. **Whooping cough** – make cabbage tea and add two teaspoons of honey to lubricate the lungs, or add apricot kernel.
3. **Frostbite** – wash the area in cabbage and green onion tea.

Carrots

Nature/Taste: cool, sweet and pungent

Actions: clears heat, detoxifies, strengthens all internal organs, benefits the eyes, relieves measles, lubricates the intestines, promotes digestion

Folk Remedies:

1. **Night blindness** – drink lukewarm carrot juice.
2. **Diphtheria with sore throat** – drink carrot top tea.
3. **Indigestion** – make carrot tea and add a teaspoon of brown sugar or maltose.
4. **Measles** – make tea from carrots, water chestnut, and cilantro to induce eruption. It goes away after completely erupting.
5. **Skin lesions or eye weakness** – make tea or juice from carrots and carrot tops.
6. **Cancer** – to prevent, cook ½ stick carrot with Chinese black mushrooms and consume daily. Also drink carrot top tea.

Cauliflower

Nature/Taste: cool and sweet

Actions: lubricates the intestines, strengthens Spleen. This vegetable is weak in action.

Conditions: constipation, weak digestion

Folk Remedies:

1. **Weak digestion** – eat lightly steamed cauliflower with bell pepper and celery.
2. **Constipation** – eat raw cauliflower in salad.

Celery

Nature/Taste: cool, sweet and slightly bitter

Actions: tonifies Kidney, stops bleeding, strengthens Spleen and Stomach, clears heat, lowers blood pressure, promotes diuresis, benefits blood

Folk Remedies:
1. **High blood pressure, hypertension** – eat celery regularly; drink three cups lightly boiled celery juice daily.
2. **Diabetes** – drink three cups lightly boiled celery juice daily. Or combine celery, yam and pumpkin to make vegetable pie.
3. **Whooping Cough** – lightly steam celery juice, add a pinch of salt, drink a warm glassful at 5am and 7pm, three days in a row.
4. **Insomnia** – drink celery and beet tops tea in the evening, two hours prior to bedtime.

Chard

Nature/Taste: neutral and sweet

Actions: clears heat, detoxifies, benefits blood

Contraindications: dysentery, boils, skin lesions

Folk Remedies:
1. **Dysentery** – make a tea from chard and dandelion greens.
2. **Boils** – mix with aloe vera juice; apply externally.

Chinese Cabbage (Napa Cabbage)

Nature/Taste: cold and sweet

Actions: clears heat, lubricates intestines, promotes diuresis and sweating

Conditions: irritability, restlessness, constipation, difficulty urinating

Folk Remedies:
1. **Constipation or difficulty urinating** – make Chinese cabbage soup.
2. **Common cold, wind-cold type** – mix Chinese cabbage and ginger, simmer into tea, and sweat.

Chinese Chive

Nature/Taste: warm and pungent

Actions: tonifies Kidneys and sexual functions, removes dampness, warms up coldness

Conditions: cold stomachache, vaginal discharge, diarrhea, bedwetting, wet dreams, absence of menstrual period

Folk Remedies:

1. **For the above conditions,** boil Chinese chive tea for 25-30 minutes.
2. **Weak sexual functions** – cook Chinese chives with black beans, black sesame seeds, walnuts, sour plums and two teaspoons honey. Make into paste and take one tablespoon, three times daily.

Cilantro Leaves (Chinese Parsley)

Nature/Taste: slightly cool,* neutral and pungent

Actions: promotes sweating, strengthens digestion, regulates Chi flow

Conditions: measles, common cold, indigestion, lack of appetite, chest and stomach fullness

Folk Remedies:

1. **Measles** – drink cilantro and mint tea to induce eruptions.
2. **Common cold of the wind-cold type** – drink cilantro and ginger tea.
3. **Common cold of the wind-heat type** – drink cilantro and mint tea.
4. **Chi stagnation** – drink cilantro and orange peel tea.

* *Cilantro seeds, or coriander, are slightly warm and beneficial to digestion.*

Collards (Collard Greens)

Nature/Taste: Pungent, bitter, cooling

Actions: regulates Chi, clears Liver heat, detoxifies, strengthens Lungs, builds strong bones

Conditions: constipation, cough, bone loss, irritability, agitation, headaches, abdominal fullness

Folk Remedies:
1. **Constipation** – alternate eating cooked collards, cabbage and beets on a daily basis
2. **Toxin buildup** – to help the liver detoxify, juice collard greens with kale, mustard greens, carrots, celery and cucumber. Drink 1-2 glasses daily.
3. **Weak bones** – make bone-building broth with organic beef bones, collard, kale, parsley and soybeans. Season to taste but stay low on sodium. Drink 1-2 cups of broth daily

Corn

Nature/Taste: cool and sweet

Actions: stops bleeding, promotes diuresis, benefits gall bladder, lowers blood pressure, clears heat, detoxifies

Conditions: difficult urination, gallstones, hepatitis, jaundice, hypertension, heart disease

Folk Remedies:
1. **Hypertension, jaundice, and gallstones** – eat corn regularly and drink fresh cornsilk tea.
2. **Detoxify and clear heat** – drink cornsilk and dandelion tea.
3. **Swelling or difficulty urinating** – drink cornsilk and pearl barley tea.
4. **High blood pressure** – drink cornsilk and chrysanthemum tea.
5. **Bloody urine** – drink corn and lotus root tea.

Cucumber

Nature/Taste: cool, sweet and bland – peels are bitter

Actions: clears heat, quenches thirst, relieves irritability, promotes diuresis

Conditions: swelling of the extremities, jaundice, diarrhea, epilepsy, sore throat, conjunctivitis

Contraindications: Eating cucumbers to excess will cause dampness. Cucumber seeds are difficult to digest.

Folk Remedies:

1. **Swelling of the extremities and jaundice** – boil tea from cucumber skins.
2. **Diarrhea** – use two teaspoons of dried cucumber meal mixed with rice porridge.
3. **Epilepsy** – boil tea from cucumber vines.
4. **Hot, scratchy, or swollen (puffy) eyes** – apply grated cucumber packs to closed eyes; leave on 20 minutes.

Daikon Radish (White Carrot)

Nature/Taste: cool, pungent and sweet

Actions: removes stagnant food, moistens lungs, resolves mucus, quenches thirst, relieves alcohol intoxication

Conditions: bronchitis, sore throat, dry cough, coughing of blood, painful urination, excess of mucus, alcohol intoxication, food retention

Contraindications: daikon radish neutralizes the effects of ginseng root; avoid consuming them together

Folk Remedies:

1. **Bronchitis or sore throat** – make daikon juice and add two drops of ginger juice, drink one cup lukewarm, three times daily.
2. **Dry cough with yellow sputum** – take warm daikon and water chestnut juice with one teaspoon honey.

3. **Burns** – apply grated daikon alone or mixed with aloe
   vera gel.
4. **Alcohol intoxication** – drink daikon juice before and
   after drinking alcoholic beverages.

Dandelion Greens

Nature/Taste: cool, bitter and slightly sweet

Actions: clears heat, detoxifies, anti-tumor, benefits liver function, promotes the flow of bile, diuretic

Conditions: toxic skin lesions, insect bites, poison oak blisters,
conjunctivitis (pink eye), Liver heat rising, beginning stages
of common cold

Folk Remedies:

1. **Toxic skin lesions** – apply crushed, fresh leaves; change
   poultice hourly.
2. **Conjunctivitis (Liver heat rising)** – make tea or juice.
3. **Common cold** – make tea from fresh dandelions (the
   whole plant), mint and licorice.
4. **Breast lumps and tumors** – apply dandelion and ginger
   poultices.

*Dandelion has been found to be extremely effective inhibiting bac-
teria, virus, and fungus. It is considered to be a natural antibiotic
similar in action to goldenseal root (Hydrastis Canadensis).*

Eggplant

Nature/Taste: cool and sweet

Actions: relieves pain, promotes urination, reduces swelling,
removes blood stagnation

Conditions: abdominal pain, dysentery, hot diarrhea, painful
urination, frostbite, canker sores, snake and scorpion bites,
anal bleeding, hepatitis, jaundice

Contraindications: not to be used for cold-type problems.

Folk Remedies:

1. **Bites** – apply fresh to absorb toxins.
2. **Jaundice and hepatitis** – eat eggplant and rice three times daily for one week.
3. **Swelling and edema** – dry the eggplant and grind to a meal; take one teaspoon in warm water three times daily.
4. **Frostbite** – soak area in eggplant tea.
5. **Canker sores** – charcoal eggplant and apply locally.

Garlic

Nature/Taste: hot and pungent

Actions: anti-viral, anti-fungal, detoxifies meat and seafood, kills worms, removes stagnant food and stagnant blood, reduces abscess

Conditions: cancer, high blood cholesterol, infections, diarrhea, dysentery, vomiting, and coughing of blood

Contraindications: not to be used with hot or dry eye disorders, mouth sores or tongue ulcers.

Folk Remedies:

1. **Vaginal infections** – boil a bulb of garlic, cool to lukewarm, then douche with the liquid.
2. **Coughing or vomiting of blood** – apply crushed, peeled, raw garlic to the soles of both feet at the depression behind the ball of the foot, also known as *rushing spring* point (Kidney 1); change the poultice every four hours.
3. **Dysentery** – mash 3-5 raw cloves, mix with warm water; drink every two hours.
4. **Vomiting** – cook together a bulb of garlic and three slices ginger; mix with a teaspoon of honey and some water.
5. **Antidote for crab poisoning** – cook garlic with crabs or other sea foods.

6. **Earache or ear infection** – put a few drops of garlic oil or juice in ear several times daily.
7. **Intestinal worms** – eat cooked garlic on an empty stomach; resume eating three hours later.

Green Beans

Nature/Taste: warm and sweet

Actions: warms Spleen and Stomach, descends Chi, tonifies Kidneys, benefits Chi

Conditions: burping, chest fullness and discomfort, whooping cough, hernia in children, chronic diarrhea, back pain due to kidney weakness

Folk Remedies:
1. **Whooping cough** – boil ½ cup green beans and 6 grams licorice in 1½ cups water; boil down to one cup and add two teaspoons honey. Drink the liquid
2. **Chronic diarrhea** – steam green beans with rice.
3. **Hernia in children** – dry-fry green beans with fennel and then grind into powder. Take ½ teaspoon, three times daily with lukewarm water. Also can be applied as a paste (green beans and fennel) to the navel with black pepper.
4. **Back pain** – make soup with green beans, black beans, azuki beans and a pinch of cinnamon powder.

Jerusalem Artichoke

Nature/Taste: sweet, neutral

Actions: tonifies Spleen and Lung Chi, regulates blood sugar, promotes digestion, replenishes Yin

Conditions: hepatitis, jaundice, diabetes, hypoglycemia, fatigue, indigestion, night sweats, frequent colds and flu

Folk Remedies:
1. **Diabetes and blood sugar imbalance** – make artichoke gratin by peeling and boiling artichoke until soft. Remove and cut into thin slices. Bake in baking pan until slightly brown. Eat artichoke gratin instead of starchy foods.
2. **Susceptibility to colds/flu** – make artichoke soup with generous amounts of garlic and onions and eat daily during flu season.

Kale

Nature/Taste: warm and slightly bitter

Actions: strengthens stomach, stops pains, promotes re-growth of tissue

Conditions: stomach or duodenal ulcers

Folk Remedies:
1. **Ulcers** – take ½ glass warm kale juice before each meal.

Lettuce

Nature/Taste: neutral and bland*

Actions: invigorates Chi, removes stagnation, reduces swelling, and softens hardening. This vegetable is mild in action.

Conditions: skin lesions, abdominal pain, breast abscess, postpartum abdominal pain due to blood stagnation

Folk Remedies:
1. **Skin lesions, insect bites, sores with pus** – apply mashed lettuce, changing poultice three times daily; and drink one cup of lukewarm lettuce juice, three times daily.
2. **Breast abscess** – make poultice and juice with dandelions. Drink the juice and apply with gauze pad externally.

* *The more bitter varieties of lettuce such as romaine or endive are cool and drying.*

Lotus Root

Nature/Taste: cool and sweet

Actions: very healing, clears heat, quenches thirst, relieves irritability, stops bleeding, strengthens stomach, promotes diuresis, cools the blood

Conditions: difficult urination, vomiting blood, nosebleed, blood in stool or urine, hypertension, gastritis, colitis

Folk Remedies:

1. **Nosebleed and hypertension** – drink lotus root juice daily.
2. **Gastritis and colitis** – drink diluted lotus root juice.
3. **Vomiting or defecating blood** – cook ½ cup of lotus root starch with ½ cup rice porridge until jelly-like consistency; consume while lukewarm.
4. **Blood in the urine** – make tea of lotus root and bamboo leaves.

Mushroom (Button)

Nature/Taste: slightly cool and sweet

Actions: induces measle eruptions, detoxifies, improves appetite, stops diarrhea, resolves phlegm, anti-tumor

Conditions: infectious hepatitis, measles, diarrhea, cough with copious mucus, low appetite

Folk Remedies:

1. **Infectious hepatitis, decrease in white cells** – eat button mushrooms in the diet or in tea.
2. **Measles** – boil tea from button mushrooms and drink one cup three times daily. Or, cook with poi and drink the broth.

Mushroom (Reishi, Ganoderma, Ling Zhi)

Nature/Taste: warm and bland

Actions: nourishes the Heart, calms the spirit, fortifies the Chi and blood

Conditions: Heart Chi deficiency, blood deficiency leading to insomnia, excessive dreaming, anxiety, restlessness, fatigue; coughs, asthma, high cholesterol, high blood pressure, coronary heart disease, chronic hepatitis, low white blood cell production

Folk Remedies:

1. **High blood pressure, high cholesterol** – Ling Zhi mushroom is usually consumed in powder or tea form on a daily routine.
2. **Chronic hepatitis** – make tea from Ling Zhi and licorice root.
3. **Chronic bronchitis** – make a tea of Ling Zhi and lily bulbs.
4. **Allergic asthma** – make tea of Ling Zhi, basil, and peppermint.
5. **Allergic rhinitis** – concentrate the Ling Zhi tea, strain through filter, then wash nose with the tea.

Mushroom (Shitake, Black)*

Nature/Taste: neutral and sweet

Actions: strengthens stomach, promotes healing, lowers blood pressure, detoxifies, anti-tumor, lowers cholesterol

Conditions: tumor, diabetes, hypertension, slow healing, high blood pressure, high cholesterol

Folk Remedies:

1. **Tumors** – boil tea from black mushrooms and drink three times daily, continuously. This can also be used as a preventative to stomach and cervical cancer. Used post surgery, this remedy is believed to prevent metastasis (spreading) of tumor cells.
2. **To clean toxins in the intestines** – soak some Chinese black mushrooms, blend with the soak water; heat like soup and take on an empty stomach. One can also add a little ginger.

* *These are also known as Chinese mushrooms.*

Mushroom (White)*

Nature/Taste: cold and sweet

Actions: clears summer heat, lowers blood pressure, anti-tumor, detoxifies

Conditions: hypertension, summer irritability, and other summer heat problems, tumors

Contraindications: white mushrooms should not be used by those with skin problems, allergies or cold stomach.

Folk Remedies:

1. **High blood cholesterol or hypertension** – use white mushrooms and cornsilk to make soup or tea regularly.
2. **Tumors** – make mushroom soup or tea daily and drink three cups daily.
3. **Summer heat problems** – eat raw mushrooms in salad.

* This is the common supermarket variety of mushroom. Seek out mushrooms that are grown without chemicals.

Mustard Greens

Nature/Taste: warm and pungent

Actions: relieves common colds, promotes urination, dissolves mucus, strengthens and lubricates intestines, ventilates Lungs, increases appetite

Conditions: difficulty urinating, coughing of blood, dysentery, sore throat, loss of voice, copious white sputum

Folk Remedies:

1. **Difficulty urinating** – make tea from fresh mustard greens and drink frequently.
2. **Coughing of blood** – make raw mustard greens juice, mix with some lukewarm water and drink gradually.
3. **Dysentery** – charcoal mustard plant roots and grind into meal. Mix six ounces of meal with water and add one teaspoon of honey; drink twice daily.

4. **Common cold (wind cold type)** – drink tea of mustard greens, cilantro and green onions and try to sweat.
5. **Copious white sputum** – drink mustard seed tea.

Onion, Leek*

Nature/Taste: warm and pungent

Actions: promotes sweating, resolves phlegm, diuretic

Conditions: common cold, acute or chronic sinus infection, upper respiratory infection, allergies, difficulty urinating, intestinal worms, certain types of boils and lesions

Folk Remedies:

1. **Common cold** – make tea from chopped onion and a few slices of fresh ginger root, or eat the onion alone.
2. **Common cold and sinus congestion in infants** – rub onion juice on baby's upper lip, under the nose, or vaporize the room with steam from onion tea.
3. **Chronic or acute sinus infection** – before bedtime rinse nasal passages with saline solution. Then extract onion juice and soak two cotton balls in it. Insert into nostrils, one at a time, and leave there for five minutes each.
4. **Cough, mucus, and upper respiratory infection** – put slices of onion over the nose like a mask and inhale the aroma for 30 minutes. Or steam the sliced onion and apply warm as a poultice to the chest area; cover to keep warm and leave on for 20-30 minutes.
5. **Difficulty urinating** – mash onion and steam it; then apply poultice to the abdomen below the navel (CV4) as a hot compress.
6. **Intestinal worms in children** – mash onion and mix with 1-2 tablespoons sesame oil and eat on an empty stomach twice a day for three consecutive days.
7. **Boils** – mash and mix with vinegar and apply to lesions.

* *The properties of onion also apply to leeks.*

Parsley

Nature/Taste: slightly warm and pungent

Actions: promotes digestion, removes stagnant food, regulates flow of Chi, induces measles eruption, diuretic

Conditions: food retention, indigestion, stomach and abdominal fullness, measles, seafood or meat poisoning

Contraindications: Over-consumption of parsley is not beneficial for the eyes.

Folk Remedies:

1. **Breast abscess** – make juice from ½ pound parsley; divide into three portions. To be taken with warm wine.
2. **Measles** – make parsley tea; drink and mix the tea with wine to be used as an external wash.
3. **Food retention, ingestion, and fullness** – make tea of parsley, hawthorn berries, daikon radish, and unsprayed, dried orange peels.

Parsley is a strong food that is eaten in small amounts. Seek naturally grown parsley, if possible.

Parsnip

Nature/Taste: warm and pungent

Actions: promotes sweating, dispels wind and dampness, relieves pain, stops bleeding (when charred)*

Conditions: common cold of the wind-cold type, headache, muscle ache, dizziness, arthritis, tetanus

Folk Remedies:

1. **Common cold (wind-cold-damp type)** – make parsnip and ginger tea.
2. **Arthritis of the wind-cold type** – combine parsnip, cinnamon, black pepper, and dry ginger to make a tea, and drink. Externally, apply either mashed, fresh jalepeno pepper or dry jalepeno mixed with some ginger tea.

* Charred parsnips used as tea are used to stop bleeding such as coughing blood or nosebleeds.

Potato

Nature/Taste: cool and sweet

Actions: relieves ulcer pain, strengthens Spleen, harmonizes Stomach, tonifies Chi, lubricates intestines, promotes diuresis, heals inflammations

Conditions: stomach and duodenal ulcers, constipation, eczema, skin lesions, swelling, small physical stature

Contraindications: Do not eat sprouted or green potatoes because they are slightly toxic.

Folk Remedies:

1. **Ulcer pain or constipation** – make raw potato juice in the blender, mix with a small amount of honey. Take two tablespoons every morning on an empty stomach. Make fresh daily.
2. **Eczema or other damp, exuding sores** – apply raw grated potato locally with gauze, change every three hours.
3. **Genital eczema** – apply raw grated potato at night; change six times; repeat for three days.
4. **Swelling** – make tea of grated potato and cucumber.

Pumpkin, Winter Squash

Winter squashes are the hard-skin varieties like acorn, butternut, buttercup, spaghetti, and kabocha

Nature/Taste: cool and sweet

Actions: dispels dampness, reduces fever, relieves pain, stabilizes hyperactive fetus, stops dysentery, benefits diabetes; the seeds kill worms and parasites

Conditions: dysentery, diabetes, ulcerations of the lower extremities, eczema, stomachache, the feeling of *steaming bones**, intestinal worms, antidote for opium

Folk Remedies:

1. **Burns** – apply fresh pumpkin alone or mixed with aloe vera gel.

2. **Lower limb ulcerations** – apply dried pumpkin meal.
3. **Intestinal worms** – take one teaspoon pumpkin seed meal three times daily on an empty stomach.
4. **Childhood vomiting** – make tea from the pumpkin stem and cap.
5. **Breast cancer** – charcoal the cap and grind to powder. Take one teaspoon of the powder in one shot of rice wine twice daily. The alcohol is a useful agent for increasing circulation and removing stagnancy. The tumor is considered to be some type of stagnant blood, Chi, or mucus.
6. **Hyperactive fetus** – take one teaspoon pumpkin ash in sweet rice porridge.
7. **Diabetes** – eat a slice of pumpkin with every meal or bake pie with pumpkin, yam, and potato.

* *The sensation of heat deep in the body as if there is "steam in the bones" is part of a condition of Yin exhaustion. Other symptoms include insomnia, irritability, flushed cheeks, heat (especially severe in late afternoon or evenings), night sweats, thirst, feverish sensation in the palms and soles.*

Scallion (Green Onion)

Nature/Taste: hot* and pungent

Actions: expels external pathogens, dispels wind and cold, induces sweating; antiviral, and antibacterial

Conditions: common cold, nasal congestion, measles, abscesses, arthritis of the *cold-type*

Contraindication: Not to be used for the *heat-type* arthritis. Not to be used for heat stages of common cold, characterized by fever, extreme thirst, and yellow sputum.

Folk Remedies:

1. **Common cold** – make tea by lightly boiling scallions for five minutes. Can also add basil.

2. **Measles** – drink scallion tea and apply raw, mashed scallions to the navel to draw out the measles.
3. **Abscesses** – mix raw scallions with egg white and apply; change poultice every four hours.
4. **Arthritis pain** – make scallion tea and soak painful area; apply mashed, cooked scallions to painful area. Scallion and clove tea is also good to drink.

* *The white part is hot, the green part is warm.*

Seaweed

Nature/Taste: cold and salty

Actions: softens hardenings, clears heat, detoxifies, benefits the thyroid gland, protects from radioactivity, benefits the lymphatic system, promotes diuresis, provides many minerals

Conditions: swollen lymph glands, goiters, cough, lung abscess with thick, yellow, odoriferous mucus, edema, beriberi, fibroid tumors, cystic breasts, nodules, lumps, cancer, low thyroid

Folk Remedies:

1. **Goiter** – make soup from dried (preferably green) orange peel, carrots, and seaweed.
2. **Lymph tuberculosis** – incorporate seaweeds into the diet for at least two months.
3. **Cough and lung abscess** – powder seaweed and mix with honey; these can be rolled into pills.
4. **Lumps, nodules, and tumors** – make tea from seaweed, peach kernel and green orange peels to take internally. Externally, make poultice of seaweed, ginger, and dandelion and apply locally.

There are many varieties of seaweed that can be easily incorporated into soups, stir-fry dishes, etc. A delicious healthful appetizer can be made with soaked hiziki or arame (looks like thin black noodles), a little soy sauce, honey, and rice vinegar. The variety of seaweed that would be the least cold is nori.

Snow Pea

Nature/Taste: cold and sweet

Actions: strengthens middle warmer, detoxifies, relieves vomiting, promotes diuresis, relieves belching, stops dysentery, promotes lactation, quenches thirst

Conditions: chronic diarrhea, dysentery, difficulty urinating, lower abdominal distention and fullness, diabetes, blocked lactation, vomiting

Folk Remedies:
1. **Diabetes** – cook snow peas, then blend juice; drink ½ cup twice daily.
2. **Hypertension** – make juice from fresh snow peas; drink ½ cup twice daily.
3. **Diarrhea** – cook snow peas in sweet rice and eat it with every meal until relieved.
4. **Poor lactation** – consume steamed snow peas frequently.

Soybean Sprouts

Nature/Taste: cool and sweet

Actions: promotes diuresis, clears heat

Conditions: food retention, Stomach heat, swelling, arthritis, spasms

Folk Remedies:
1. **Hypertension** – boil tea for four hours; drink lukewarm, daily over a period of one month.
2. **Warts** – eat only steamed soybean sprouts for three days consecutively without eating anything else.

Spinach

Nature/Taste: cool and sweet

Actions: strengthens all organs, lubricates intestines, promotes urination, ventilates the chest, quenches thirst

Conditions: constipation, thirst, tightness in chest, inability to urinate, night blindness, alcohol intoxication, diabetes

Contraindications: not to be used with diarrhea or a history of kidney stones. Also, spinach does not mix well with tofu or dairy products due to the unhealthy combination that results from the oxalic acid in the spinach and the high calcium foods. This can lead to crystallized stones in the kidneys, if one is so predisposed.

Folk Remedies:

1. **Acute Conjunctivitis** – simmer spinach and chrysanthemum flowers; drink the liquid.
2. **Night blindness** – make fresh spinach juice, drink one cup twice daily.
3. **Diabetes** – boil tea from spinach and chicken gizzard, drink one cup three times daily.
4. **Constipation, urinary obstruction, headache** – drink spinach soup.

Squash, Summer (Zucchini)

Summer squash includes all the soft skin varieties. See "Pumpkin" for properties of winter squash

Nature/Taste: cool and sweet

Actions: clears heat, detoxifies, promotes diuresis, quenches thirst, relieves restlessness

Conditions: skin lesions, difficulty urinating, edema, summer heat, irritability, thirst

Contraindications: not to be used in beriberi or scabies.

Folk Remedies:

1. *Burns* – preserve cut up squash until it becomes liquid (usually 6-12 months) and apply the liquid to the burn.
2. *Edema in the extremities or the abdomen* – cook squash with vinegar until soggy and eat on empty stomach or make tea from squash skin.

3. *Summer heat and irritability* – eat squash as a salad.
4. *Jaundice* – drink tea made from squash skin, one cup three times daily.

Sweet Potato, Yam

Nature/Taste: neutral and sweet

Actions: strengthens Spleen and Stomach function, tonifies Chi, clears heat, detoxifies, increases the production of milk

Conditions: bloody stools, diarrhea, constipation, jaundice, edema, ascites, night blindness, diabetes, breast abscess, boils, skin lesions

Contraindications: Overeating sweet potatoes will cause gas, heartburn, indigestion, abdominal distention and acid regurgitation.

Folk Remedies:

1. **Night blindness** – cook yam or sweet potato with animal liver (preferably goat).
2. **Jaundice** – cook yam soup with squash and pearl barley.
3. **Shingles and breast abscess** – apply grated, raw yam locally or mix in a pinch of borax.
4. **Eczema (particularly genital eczema)** – make tea with sweet potato and a pinch of salt and bathe the area. Sprinkle afterwards with natural talcum powder.
5. **Poison insect bites** – mash yam or sweet potato with honey and apply.
6. **Cirrhosis of the liver and accompanying edema in the abdomen** – apply to the navel a mixture of mashed sweet potato and brown sugar; change hourly.
7. **Diabetes** – cook soup with winter melon.
8. **Bloody stools** – mix sweet potato powder or yam powder with honey.

Taro Root

Nature/Taste: neutral, sweet and pungent

Actions: clears heat, reduces swelling, benefits Spleen, regulates digestive system

Conditions: swollen lymph glands, nodules, goiters, externally for pain from tendonitis, sprains, traumas, snake bites, bee stings

Contraindications: If you eat too much, taro root can cause food retention and stomach pains. Externally, can cause allergic reaction in some people; an antidote for this would be to apply fresh ginger juice. Also, it is slightly toxic raw.

Folk Remedies:

1. **Externally for infections such as pleurisy, peritonitis, appendicitis, joint pain, sciatica, back pain, arthritis** – mix peeled taro root and ginger together with flour and water until a paste is formed. Apply to the affected area and cover with a cloth. During winter, heat up the paste and apply. Change daily and always apply a fresh mixture.
2. **Snake bite, bees sting, and bug bites** – mash taro root with a pinch of salt and apply locally.
3. **Blisters that contain fluid** – charcoal taro to ash, mix with sesame oil and apply to blister.
4. **Swollen lymph glands, nodules, scrofula, goiter, and tuberculosis** – dry taro root, grind to powder, then take equal parts of water chestnuts and jellyfish and boil into tea. Take the liquid and mix with the taro root powder; roll into pills the size of mung beans, take two tablespoons of pills three times daily with warm water.

Turnip

Nature/Taste: warm, sweet, bitter and pungent

Actions: regulates Chi, dries dampness, promotes digestion, transforms phlegm

Conditions: indigestion, bloating, excess gas, wet cough, diarrhea, heaviness

Folk Remedies:

1. **Indigestion and gas** – dice 1 turnip and boil in 4 cup of water with 3-4 pieces of tangerine or orange peel and 5 slices of fresh ginger root for 30 minutes. Strain and drink 3 cups of liquid daily right after each meal.
2. **Diarrhea and malaise** – make steamed turnip cake by grating 2 turnips, mix with 1 cup barley flour and water, season to taste and put in cake pan and steam for an hour in a double boiler. Eat 1/4 slice each day.
3. **Productive cough** – juice raw turnip, and mix with honey and warm water. Drink 2-3 cups a day.

Water Chestnut

Nature/Taste: cold and sweet

Actions: clears heat and stops bleeding

Conditions: dry cough due to heat in the lungs with thick, tenacious mucus, jaundice, bloody stool, excessive uterine bleeding, antidote for lead and copper poisoning

Folk Remedies:

1. **Bloody stools** – juice fresh water chestnuts and mix with equal amount of rice wine and drink three times a day on an empty stomach. Results should be seen within three days.
2. **Excess uterine bleeding** – charcoal the water chestnuts, powder them and take with rice wine.
3. **Bronchitis, pneumonia, cough** – make tea from fresh water chestnuts and honeysuckle flowers; drink 3-5 cups daily.
4. **Lead and copper poisoning** – consume daily 1 pound of fresh water chestnuts with ¼ pound of peach kernels.

Watercress

Nature/Taste: cool and bitter

Actions: clears heat, quenches thirst, lubricates lungs, promotes diuresis

Conditions: thirst, irritability, restlessness, sore and dry throat, cough with yellow sputum

Contraindications: not to be used in cases of diarrhea.

Folk Remedies:
1. **Thirst, irritability, and sore throat** – drink fresh, raw watercress juice.
2. **Cough** – boil tea from watercress and apricot kernels (or almonds). Remove the apex of the apricot kernel, which is toxic. Drink one cup three times daily.

Winter Melon

Nature/Taste: cool, sweet and bland

Actions: clears heat, detoxifies, promotes urination, quenches thirst, relieves irritability, dispels dampness, antidote for seafood poisoning

Conditions: boils, skin lesions, ascites (edema in the abdomen), difficult urination, heatstroke

Folk Remedies:
1. **Hives** – make tea of winter melon skin and drink.
2. **Chronic nephritis** – cook winter melon with poi, no salt added.
3. **Difficulty urinating** – drink the fresh juice with honey.
4. **Heatstroke** – make winter melon soup and drink three times daily.
5. **Promote lactation** – cook winter melon rind with trout.
6. **Summer heat with continuous high fever** – make tea from winter melon rind and grapefruit seeds (remove shells or crush seeds) and drink constantly.

Yam (see **Sweet Potato**)

Fruits

Apple

Nature/Taste: cool, sweet and slightly sour

Actions: strengthens Heart, tonifies Chi, quenches thirst, reduces dryness, alleviates thirst, lubricates lungs, resolves mucus

Conditions: dry throat, dehydration, indigestion, hypertension, constipation, chronic diarrhea

Folk Remedies:

1. **Constipation** – eat a fresh apple on an empty stomach.
2. **Indigestion** – eat an apple after each meal.
3. **Diarrhea** – take two teaspoons of powdered, dried apple three times daily on an empty stomach.
4. **Cough with yellow sputum** – drink apple juice.
5. **Hypertension** – eat three apples a day.
6. **General cleansing** – fast one day a week on apples, apple juice, and beet top tea. The apples contain pectin that acts as a broom in our intestines.

For problems of a cold nature, bake the apples to decrease their cooling properties.

Apricot

Nature/Taste: slightly cool, sweet and sour

Actions: regenerates body fluids, clears heat, detoxifies, quenches thirst

Conditions: dehydration, thirst, cough

Contraindications: too much injures bones and tendons and produces mucus; in children this can cause skin rashes. Not good to eat too many during pregnancy.

Folk Remedies:

1. **Summer thirst and dehydration** – eat fresh apricots (no more than 5-10).

2. **Cough** – make tea from one teaspoon of ground apricot kernels, adding a bit of honey. The inner kernel of the apricot seed is used to ventilate lungs, descend rebellious Chi, lubricate intestines, relieve constipation, relieve cough and asthma. One should remove the apex of the kernel, which is toxic.

Avocado

Nature/Taste: sweet, cool

Actions: nourishes Yin and blood; moistens lungs, skin and intestines

Conditions: anemia, palpitations, dry skin, constipation/dry stools, dry cough, diabetes, menopausal hot flashes

Contraindications: diarrhea

Folk Remedies:
1. **Anemia and palpitations** – eat 1/2 an avocado daily for one month. Retest to monitor progress.
2. **Constipation and dry skin** – make a shake with 1/2 avocado, 1 banana, 1/2 cup of yogurt with 1 cup of almond milk. Drink for breakfast.
3. **Menopausal hot flashes** – make avocado ice cream with soymilk by blending 1 avocado with I cup of soymilk until smooth and put in freezer. Eat one scoop each day until hot flashes abate.

Banana

Nature/Taste: cold and sweet

Actions: clears heat, lubricates lungs, lubricates intestines, lowers blood pressure, helps alleviate alcohol intoxication

Conditions: constipation, thirst, cough, hemorrhoids, hypertension, alcohol intoxication

Contraindications: not to be used in cold conditions.

Folk Remedies:
1. **Hemorrhoids and constipation** – eat a banana every day on an empty stomach.

2. **Hypertension** – drink organic banana peel tea.
3. **Cough** – cook banana with a bit of sugar. Note, this may not be appropriate of Americans who already consume about 120 pounds of sugar a year. If honey is substituted, do not cook the honey.

Blueberry

Nature/Taste: sour, sweet, warm

Actions: tonifies Kidneys, nourishes blood, astringes Chi, slows aging process

Conditions: poor concentration, memory decline, kidney weakness, frequent urination, anemia

Folk Remedies:
1. **Poor concentration/ADD:** incorporate 1/4 cup of either fresh or frozen blueberries into breakfast daily for 2-4 weeks
2. **Memory decline:** make trail mix of equal portions of dried blueberries, walnuts, pine nuts, goji/lycii berries and pumpkin seeds
3. **Anemia and Kidney weakness:** mix together dried blueberries, raisins and figs and eat a handful

Cantaloupe

Nature/Taste: cold and sweet

Actions: clears heat, quenches thirst, relieves summer heat problems, eases urination

Conditions: summer heat thirst, lung abscess, irritability

Contraindications: not for cold conditions, history of coughing or vomiting blood, diarrhea, ulcers, heart disease, or weak stomach. Melons may upset stomach if eaten with other food and should be eaten alone.

Folk Remedies:
1. **To induce vomiting** – take dried, ground cantaloupe seeds in warm water.

Cherry

Nature/Taste: warm and sweet

Actions: benefits skin and overall body, rejuvenates, strengthens Spleen, stimulates appetite, stops dysentery and diarrhea, quenches thirst, regenerates fluids, stops involuntary seminal emissions, prolongs life

Conditions: measles, burns, diarrhea, dysentery, thirst, premature ejaculation

Contraindications: eaten in excess will cause nausea, vomiting, skin lesions and cause a person to feel hot. This injures the bones and tendons.

Folk Remedies:
1. **Measles** – drink fresh warmed cherry juice.
2. **Burns** – apply locally.
3. **Enlarged thyroid or goiter** – soak cherry pits in vinegar until they disintegrate, then apply locally.
4. **Hernia pain** – fry cherry pits with vinegar, mash to powder; take one teaspoon per dose.

Chinese Dates (Red or Black Jujube)

Nature/Taste: neutral* and sweet

Actions: strengthens Spleen, tonifies Yin, nourishes the body, tonifies blood, lubricates lungs, stops coughs, stops diarrhea, harmonizes within the body or within an herb formula. For example, dates and licorice can reduce the harshness of a food or herb and unite the combination into action.

Conditions: Yin deficiency, weak digestion, cough, night sweats, weakness, anemia, blood in urine, diarrhea, bruises, nervous hysteria

Contraindications: too much creates mucus, distended stomach, and is hard on the teeth.

Folk Remedies:
1. **Blood in urine** – drink red date tea.

2. **Spontaneous sweating** – boil tea from ten red dates and ten preserved plums.

* *Black dates are slightly warming.*

Chinese Prune

These prunes are made from half ripened plums and have a sour flavor. They are more beneficial therapeutically than the sweet variety that is made from fully ripened plums.

Nature/Taste: warm and sour

Actions: astringes intestines, stops diarrhea, kills worms, stops cough, consolidates the Lungs, quenches thirst, promotes body fluids. The sweet prunes quench thirst, promote body fluids, and moisten the intestines.

Folk Remedies:
1. **Dysentery** – for both prevention (as before a trip to a third-world country) and treatment, brew prune tea and take before meals on an empty stomach.
2. **Intestinal worms** – make tea with prunes and black pepper.
3. **Fish bones stuck in the throat** – brew concentrated prune tea and add an equal part of rice vinegar; drink slowly. The herb clematis, powdered and mixed with rice vinegar could be given in an emergency, to dissolve a fish bone.
4. **Summer heat irritability** – drink prune juice.

Coconut

Nature/Taste: warm* and sweet

Actions: strengthens the body, reduces swelling, stops bleeding, kills worms, activates heart function

Conditions: weakness, nosebleeds, intestinal or skin worms

Folk Remedies:
1. **Worms** – every morning on an empty stomach, drink the juice and eat the meat of ½ coconut; wait three hours before eating anything else.

2. **Edema due to weak heart** – drink plenty of coconut juice.

* *The milk inside of the coconut is neutral and sweet.*

Cranberry

Nature/Taste: Sour, cooling

Actions: promotes urination, relieves painful urination, strengthens Kidneys and reproductive system

Conditions: frequent urination, painful burning urination, incontinence, Kidney weakness, kidney stones, infertility

Contraindications: gastric acid reflux

Folk Remedies:

1. **Bladder infection** – drink 1 cup cranberry juice (preferably unsweetened and diluted) along with 1,000 mg. vitamin C every 3-4 hours a day. Drink an additional 5-6 cups of water daily. If symptoms persist beyond 3 days or lower back pain begins, see your doctor immediately.
2. **Kidney stones and bladder infection prevention** – drink 1 cup of unsweetened cranberry juice along with 8 glasses of water daily. Avoid high oxalate foods such as spinach, chard and beet greens.
3. **Infertility** – make a fertility-enhancing trail mix consisting of equal parts of dried cranberries, walnuts, sesame seeds, longan fruit, and cashews.

Fig

Nature/Taste: cool and sweet

Actions: clears heat, lubricates lungs and intestines, stop diarrhea

Conditions: dry cough, dry throat, Lung heat, constipation, indigestion, hemorrhoids, prolapse of the rectum

Folk Remedies:

1. **Lung-heat symptoms** – make tea from figs (preferably fresh).

2. **Hemorrhoids** – bathe area in fig tea.
3. **Asthma** – blend fig juice and drink three times daily.
4. **Hernia** – drink fig and fennel tea.

Goji Berry (Lycium Berry or Gou Qi Zi)

Nature/Taste: sweet, sour, neutral

Actions: nourishes blood and Yin, strengthens the Lungs, benefits Liver and Kidney, improves vision, stop cough

Conditions: vision decline, anemia, lower back pain, impotence, tinnitus, chronic dry cough, diabetes

Contraindication: fevers, common cold and flu

Folk Remedies:

1. **Vision decline or diabetes** – make vision enhancing trail mix with equal parts of dried goji berry, plums, sunflower seeds, pistachios and pine nuts. Eat a small handful daily as a snack.
2. **Anemia** – traditional Chinese blood tonic recipe calls for making chicken soup with 1/4 cup of dried goji berries, red jujube date, dang gui root, astragalus root and fresh ginger root. Eat daily until anemia improves.
3. **Tinnitus** – make tea by boiling 1/4 cup dried goji berries and 1/2 cup chrysanthemum blossoms in 4 cups of water for 15 minutes. Strain immediately and drink 3 cups daily.

Grape

Nature/Taste: warm, sweet and sour

Actions: very tonifying (particularly the red or purple varieties), nourishes blood, strengthens bones and tendons, tonifies Chi, harmonizes Stomach, promotes diuresis, relieves irritability

Conditions: cold type arthritis, tendonitis, painful urination, hepatitis, jaundice, anemia, flu

Contraindications: Wine should not be combined with fatty foods because it can result in phlegm and heat that rises to the heart and can cause strokes and heart attacks. Also, excessive consumption of grapes leads to constipation or diarrhea.

Folk Remedies:
1. **Anemia** – eat raisins.
2. **Arthritis (cold type) and tendonitis** – make grape vine tea and add some wine. The moderate use of wine can be of benefit in cold environments and cold conditions.
3. **Hepatitis and jaundice** – make grape tea.
4. **Flu** – drink grape juice.

Grapefruit

Nature/Taste: cold, sweet and sour

Actions: strengthens stomach, aids digestion, circulates Chi, detoxifies alcohol intoxication

Conditions: decreased appetite, weak digestion, stomach fullness, alcohol intoxication, dry cough

Contraindication: grapefruit and grapefruit juice can interfere with certain medications including anti-hypertensives, statin drugs, antihistamines, and drugs that decrease anxiety. Consult with your doctor or pharmacist before consuming grapefruit if you are taking any medications.

Folk Remedies:
1. **Dry cough** – cook four grapefruit slices with either pork or cabbage.
2. **Chronic cough** – make tea from about 20 grapefruit seeds, adding a bit of honey; drink three times daily.
3. **Jaundice and stomach distention** – char and powder grapefruit peel;* take a teaspoon with warm water three times daily.
4. **Gastritis or inflammation of the stomach** – make tea from aged grapefruit peel, green tea leaves, and two slices of fresh ginger; drink all day.
5. **Frostbite** – wash or soak area in grapefruit peel tea.

* *Grapefruit peel is warming and can be used to dispel cold, regulate Chi, aid digestion, dry dampness, resolve sputum, and aid wind-cold cough, stomach distention and scratchy throat. Make tea from the dried peel.*

Hawthorn Berry

Nature/Taste: slightly warm, sweet and sour

Actions: strengthens Spleen, removes stagnant food, invigorates blood, dissolves sputum, relieves stagnant Chi, aids digestion

Conditions: food stagnation (especially meat), bloody stools, abdominal pain, absence of menstruation due to blood stagnation, poor appetite, hypertension, high cholesterol

Folk Remedies:
1. **Child with no appetite** – give berries or tea daily.
2. **Hypertension** – drink tea daily.

Lemon, Limes

Nature/Taste: cool and sour

Actions: regenerates body fluids, harmonizes Stomach, regulates Chi, quenches thirst, benefits Liver

Conditions: sore throat, dry mouth, stomach distention, cough

Folk Remedies:
1. **Hypertension** – make tea from one peeled lemon, ten fresh water chestnuts, and 2½ cups of water; drink once daily.
2. **Sore throat** – drink lemon tea with honey.
3. **Regulate Chi, benefit Liver** – squeeze a half lemon in warm water and drink every morning.

Litchi Fruit (Lychee)

Nature/Taste: warm, sweet and astringent

Actions: nourishes blood, calms spirit, soothes Liver, regulates Chi

Conditions: hernia, weak and deficient conditions, irritability, restless heart

Contraindications: over-consumption can lead to nosebleed, feverish sensation, thirst. Not to be used in any type of heat condition.

Folk Remedies:
1. **Weak conditions, blood deficiency** – take dried litchi and black jujube date (seven of each) and boil tea; drink daily.
2. **Bedwetting** – eat ten dried litchis daily.
3. **Nausea, vomiting, burping, and belching** – take dried litchi with the kernel, charcoal powder and take with warm water.
4. **Bleeding after birth or abortion** – take seven dried litchis, mash and boil with two cups of water; reduce to one cup, drink three times daily until the bleeding stops.
5. **Hernia** – take litchi kernel, bake and grind to powder; take one teaspoon on an empty stomach daily. Or, grind the litchi kernel, mix with rice wine and take every morning on an empty stomach.

Loquat

Nature/Taste: neutral, sweet and sour

Actions: lubricates dryness, stops cough, harmonizes Stomach, descends rebellious Chi, calms the Liver

Conditions: dry mouth, thirst, irritability, dry cough, nausea, vomiting

Folk Remedies:
1. **Vomiting and nausea** – boil loquats to make tea.
2. **Cough** – eat fresh loquats.

Mango

Nature/Taste: neutral, sweet and sour

Actions: regenerates body fluids, stops cough, stops thirst, strengthens stomach

Conditions: cough, thirst, poor digestion, enlarged prostate, nausea

Contraindications: Overeating mangos can cause itching or skin eruptions.

Folk Remedies:
1. **Enlarged prostate** – boil mango peel and seed into tea.
2. **Weak digestion** – drink mango juice.

Mulberry

Nature/Taste: slightly cold and sweet

Actions: quenches thirst, detoxifies, nourishes blood, tonifies Kidneys, lubricates lungs, relieves constipation, calms the spirit, promotes urination

Conditions: thirst, irritability, dry mouth, diabetes, anemia, constipation, back pain due to Kidney weakness, alcohol intoxication, lymph node enlargement, blurred vision

Folk Remedies:
1. **Cough** – take two teaspoons of mulberry syrup twice daily. The syrup can be made by cooking mulberries on low flame until they dissolve, then adding honey and cooking down to a thick syrup.
2. **Constipation** – drink mulberry juice.
3. **Insomnia** – boil mulberry tea and drink ½ cup.

Orange

Nature/Taste: cool, sweet and sour

Actions: lubricates lungs, resolves mucus, increases appetite, strengthens Spleen, quenches thirst, promotes body fluids

Conditions: thirst, dehydration, stagnant Chi, hernia

Folk Remedies:
1. **Cough with copious mucus** – cook the orange and eat it.
2. **Stuck mucus, stagnant Chi, chest fullness or distention**– make tea from unsprayed, dried orange peel.*
3. **Chi stagnation, prostate enlargement and hernia** – make tea from orange seeds.

* Orange peel is warm, bitter and pungent, and is used to invigorate the movement of Chi and dry dampness.

Papaya

Nature/Taste: neutral, sweet and sour

Actions: strengthens Stomach and Spleen, aids digestion, clears summer heat, lubricates lungs, stops cough, aids irritability, kills worms, increases milk production

Conditions: cough, indigestion, stomachache, eczema, skin lesions, intestinal worms

Folk Remedies:
1. **Increasing lactation** – put fresh papaya in fish soup.
2. **Cough** – peel and steam papaya, then add honey.
3. **Stomachache and indigestion** – cook papaya and eat with or after meals.
4. **Intestinal worms** – sun dry green papaya, powder, and take two teaspoons on an empty stomach every morning.
5. **Skin lesions** – apply fresh papaya.

Dried papaya is warm, sweet and sour. It is used to invigorate and activate the channels, aid digestion, and resolve dampness.

Peach

Nature/Taste: very cool, sweet and slightly sour

Actions: lubricates lungs, clears heat, aids diabetes, promotes body fluids, induces sweating

Conditions: diabetes, dry cough, intestinal worms, vaginitis

Contraindications: not to be used with damp and cold conditions.

Folk Remedies:

1. **Inducing sweating or killing worms** – drink peach leaf tea.
2. **Promoting blood circulation** – make tea from the innermost seed, the kernel.
3. **Dry cough** – eat fresh peaches.
4. **Vaginitis** – douche with peach leaf tea.

Pear Apple (Asian Pear)

Nature/Taste: cold and sweet

Actions: regenerates body fluids, quenches thirst, calms the Heart, lubricates lungs, relieves restlessness, promotes urination, clears heat, detoxifies, lubricates the throat, dissolves mucus, descends Chi and stops cough

Conditions: cough due to heat in the lungs, excess mucus, irritability, thirst, dry throat, hoarse throat, retina pain, constipation, difficult urination, skin lesions, alcohol intoxication

Contraindications: not to be used with cold stomach and Spleen, manifesting as cold extremities or diarrhea. Also, not to be used by pregnant women, or in cases of anemia.

Folk Remedies:

1. **Cough and bronchitis** – core the pear and steam it; eat 3-4 times daily. Pear can also be cooked with scallions.
2. **Cough with yellow phlegm** – core pear, and fill with 3 grams powdered fritillaria bulb (Chuan Bei Mu) and a little rock sugar or brown sugar; steam about 30 minutes and eat completely.
3. **Acute voice loss** – peel and juice 2-3 pears, adding two teaspoons of honey.
4. **Whooping cough** – core the pear and insert ½ gram of ephedra; steam, then remove the herb and eat the pear.
5. **Nausea, belching** – core the pear and insert 10-15 cloves; steam, then remove the cloves and eat the pear.

6. **Alcohol intoxication** – drink pear juice or tea to prevent hangover.

Domestic pear has the same properties as the Asian pear but is milder.

Persimmon

Nature/Taste: cool, sweet and astringent

Actions: lubricates lungs, stops cough with heat, dissolves sputum, strengthens Spleen, stops diarrhea, quenches thirst, clears heat

Conditions: pain in the throat due to heat, cough, thirst, vomiting blood, dysentery, alcohol intoxication

Contraindications: Do not eat persimmons along with crabs, because the combination produces extreme diarrhea.

Folk Remedies:

1. **Vomiting or coughing blood** – cook a partially ripened persimmon in rice wine for ten minutes; eat the persimmon. Another remedy is to take dried, charred persimmon powder in warm water.
2. **Bleeding ulcers and lower intestinal bleeding** – take dried, charred, powdered persimmon in warm water (about a tablespoon of the powder).
3. **Hypertension** – drink three glasses of unripened persimmon juice daily.
4. **Nausea and vomiting** – add dried persimmon to water to make a mush, steam it and take two tablespoons three times daily for 3-4 days or until condition ceases. Cloves could be a good addition; or make persimmon cap and cloves tea.
5. **Alcohol intoxication** – drink persimmon juice or tea.
6. **Ulcerated skin lesions** – apply a combination of charred persimmon powder and black pepper.

Pineapple

Nature/Taste: warm, sweet and sour

Actions: aids digestion, stops diarrhea, dispels summer heat

Conditions: heatstroke, irritability, thirst, indigestion, diarrhea

Contraindications: Pineapples are slightly toxic; this can be neutralized by washing with salt water. Pineapple is also said to generate dampness, so not to be used in those conditions.

Folk Remedies:
1. **Heat stroke and irritability** – drink fresh pineapple juice.
2. **Nephritis (kidney inflammation)** – make tea from peeled pineapple and reed roots; drink freely throughout the day.
3. **Bronchitis** – boil tea of pineapple and add honey.
4. **Dysentery** – boil tea of pineapple.

Plum

Nature/Taste: slightly warm, sweet and sour

Actions: stimulates appetite, aids digestion, regulates body fluids, stops thirst, softens or soothes the Liver, removes stagnation of Chi, removes the feeling of *steaming bones* (see pg. 44)

Conditions: dehydration, thirst, Chi stagnation, erratic energy flow, poor digestion, dysentery

Contraindication: Too many plums are not good for the teeth.

Folk Remedies:
1. **Dysentery** – drink plum skin tea.

Pomegranate

Nature/Taste: Sour, astringent, slightly warming

Actions: Astringes intestines, stops diarrhea, nourishes blood, Yin and fluids

Conditions: chronic diarrhea, anemia, incontinence, nocturnal emission, thirst, diabetes

Contraindications: common cold, flu, constipation

Folk Remedies:

1. **Diabetes and excess thirst** – make fresh pomegranate and cucumber juice with a juicer and drink 1 glass daily. Don't drink sweetened pomegranate juice.
2. **Incontinence** – mix equal portions of pomegranate and cranberry juices and drink 2 glasses daily
3. **Diarrhea** – ground dried pomegranates into powder and take 1 tsp with warm water 3 times a day. Alternatively, take pure pomegranate capsules instead.

Raspberry

Nature/Taste: slightly warm, sweet and sour

Actions: tonifies Liver and Kidneys, astringes essence, astringes urination, brightens the eyes

Conditions: Kidney and Liver deficiency, blurry vision, spermatorrhea, involuntary seminal emission, frequent urination

Folk Remedies:

1. **Impotence and involuntary seminal emission** – take dry raspberries, charcoal and grind to powder; take three teaspoons every night before bed with some rice wine.
2. **Bedwetting or frequent urination** – take charcoaled, raspberry powder, make tea and drink before bedtime every night.
3. **Eczema, skin lesions, and fungus conditions** – boil fresh raspberries to a concentrate; wash area with this.

Raspberry leaf is very strengthening to the female system, and can be used throughout pregnancy, as well as other phases of a woman's life. It is generally taken as tea.

Strawberry

Nature/Taste: cool, sweet and sour

Actions: lubricates lungs, promotes body fluids, strengthens Spleen, detoxifies in alcohol intoxication

Conditions: dry cough, sore throat, difficult urination, food retention, lack of appetite

Folk Remedies:

1. **Dry cough** – mash strawberries with brown sugar; steam and eat three times daily.
2. **Dry throat, thirst, hoarse voice, sore throat** – take one glass fresh strawberry juice twice daily.
3. **Difficult urination** – mash fresh strawberries, add cold water; drink three times daily.
4. **Lack of appetite, food retention, abdominal distention and pain** – eat five strawberries before each meal.

Tangerine

Nature/Taste: warm, sweet and sour

Actions: carminative, opens the channels, strengthens the stomach, stops cough

Conditions: nausea, vomiting, cough, excess white or clear mucus, chest tightness, rib pain

Folk Remedies:

1. **Nausea, vomiting, stomach discomfort** – make tea from unsprayed tangerine peels,* fresh ginger root and cardamom seeds.
2. **Chest fullness, pain in ribs** – use tangerine fruit combined with rice wine and water to make a tea.
3. **Hernia, testicular pain** – roast equal parts of tangerine seeds and fennel seeds; grind to powder. Take 3-6 grams with warm sake before bed.

* *Tangerine peel is warm, pungent and bitter; carminative, arrests cough, strengthens stomach and resolves phlegm.*

Tomato

Nature/Taste: slightly cool, sweet and sour

Actions: promotes body fluids, quenches thirst, strengthens stomach, aids digestion, cools blood, clears heat, detoxifies, calms the Liver, removes stagnant food

Conditions: Liver heat rising, hypertension, bloodshot eyes, dehydration, indigestion due to low stomach acid, food retention, kidney infection

Folk Remedies:

1. **Hypertension and eye hemorrhage** – eat two raw tomatoes on an empty stomach, every day for one month; also avoid spicy foods.
2. **Kidney disease** – eat at least one raw tomato per day.
3. **Indigestion and food retention** – eat half or one whole fresh tomato after meals.

Watermelon

Nature/Taste: cold and sweet

Actions: quenches thirst, relieves irritability, dispels summer heat problems, promotes diuresis, detoxifies

Conditions: sores, dry mouth, summer heat irritability, bloody dysentery, jaundice, edema, difficult urination

Contraindication: Not to be used in cold conditions, with weak stomach or with excessive urination

Folk Remedies:

1. **Edema from nephritis** – boil tea from the rind and the inner portion.
2. **Jaundice** – boil tea from the rind and red beans.
3. **Fluid in the abdomen** – make tea from the skins of watermelon, squash, and winter melon.
4. **Constipation** – boil tea from watermelon seeds or grind into meal and take with warm water.

Grains

Amaranth

Nature/Taste: sweet, bitter, warming

Actions: tonifies Chi, nourishes blood, strengthens Spleen, reduces dampness, calms spirit

Conditions: fatigue, dizziness, anemia, diarrhea, bloating, insomnia, anxiety

Folk Remedies:

1. **Fatigue or anemia** – substitute amaranth, which is rich in iron, for other grains in your diet.
2. **Diarrhea or bloating** – avoid all gluten-containing grains such as wheat, barley, rye and oats. Cook amaranth with brown rice and use them as a staple.
3. **Anxiety or insomnia** – toast 1/4 cup amaranth in oven until slightly brown, remove and steep in a cup of hot water for 5 minutes and sip for immediate relief of anxiety or before bedtime for insomnia.

Barley

Nature/Taste: sweet, cooling

Actions: tonifies Chi, promotes urination, reduces dampness, soothes irritation in the digestive system and urinary tract

Conditions: indigestion, bloating, diarrhea, swelling, painful urination, fatigue

Folk Remedies:

1. **Indigestion, bloating and gas pain:** boil 1/2 cup of barley with 5 slices of fresh ginger root in 4 cups of water for 30 minutes. Strain, and drink 3 cups daily.
2. **Fatigue and swelling during summer heat:** toast barley; combine with an equal amount of green tea. Steep 1 tbsp. of mixture in 1 cup hot water and drink 2 cups a day.

3. **Painful urination:** boil 1/4 cup barley, 1/4 cup mung beans and a handful of corn silk in 4 cups of water for 30 minutes. Strain and drink 3 cups for up to 3 days. If symptoms persist, see your doctor immediately.
4. **Detoxification:** take 2 tbsp. barley greens powder in 1 cup of water on empty stomach daily for cleansing of bowels and general detoxification.

Buckwheat

Nature/Taste: neutral and sweet

Actions: descends Chi, strengthens stomach, stops dysentery, lowers blood pressure, strengthens blood vessels

Conditions: chronic diarrhea, dysentery, spontaneous sweating, hypertension, skin lesions

Folk Remedies:
1. **Skin lesions** – boil buckwheat tea and wash area with it. Or, roast buckwheat, grind to powder and mix with rice vinegar to make a paste; then apply to area.
2. **Leukorrhea and chronic diarrhea** – grind roasted buckwheat, mix with warm water and take two teaspoons twice daily.
3. **High blood pressure** – make tea from buckwheat and lotus root.
4. **Hemorrhoids** – mix rooster bile with buckwheat meal and roll in pill form. Take one teaspoon of pills twice daily.

Cornmeal

Nature/Taste: neutral and sweet

Actions: tonifies Chi, strengthens the Stomach and Spleen, benefits the Heart, diuretic, stimulates the flow of bile

Conditions: weak digestion, heart disease, high blood pressure, edema, gallstones

Folk Remedies:

1. **Weak digestion** – make a soupy porridge with corn-meal. This is an easy to digest meal for recovery from the flu or cold.
2. **Edema, difficult urination, hypertension** – eat corn-meal regularly and drink cornsilk tea.

Fresh corn and cornsilk are cooling and more diuretic than dried cornmeal.

Kamut

Nature/Taste: sweet, cooling

Actions: tonifies Chi, strengthens Spleen and Stomach, regulates Chi, reduces bloating

Conditions: low appetite, abdominal distention and fullness, diarrhea, muscle fatigue, underweight

Folk Remedies:

1. **Underweight** – incorporate kamut into diet as a daily staple
2. **Muscle fatigue** – eat kamut cereal 1/2 hour before exercising or exerting muscle
3. **Abdominal distention** – cook kamut with tangerine peel, fennel and ginger.

Kamut, as well as spelt, is an ancient cousin of wheat that tends to create less allergic reactions, but those sensitive to gluten should avoid kamut.

Millet

Nature/Taste: cool and sweet

Actions: stops vomiting, relieves diarrhea, consolidates or astringes the stomach and intestines, clears heat, promotes urination, soothes morning sickness

Folk Remedies:

1. **Morning sickness and vomiting** – eat millet porridge as a regular staple; may add fresh ginger.

2. **Diarrhea** – roast millet until aromatic; eat ½ cup three times daily.
3. **Obstructed urination** – boil tea from millet and add ½ teaspoon brown sugar.
4. **Diabetes** – steam millet with yams and jujube dates.

Oats

Nature/Taste: warm and sweet

Actions: strengthens Spleen, tonifies and regulates Chi, harmonizes Stomach, carminative, stops lactation (sprouted form only)

Conditions: lack of appetite, indigestion, abdominal distention and fullness, dysentery, swelling

Folk Remedies:
1. **Stop lactation** – boil sprouted oats or sprouted barley tea and drink one cups three times daily. Or, use barley malt as a sweetener in the diet.
2. **Swelling** – cook oats and azuki or mung beans to a mush.
3. **Postpartum urinary and bowel obstruction** – roast sprouted oats, grind into meal, take two teaspoons three times a day with lukewarm water.
4. **Hepatitis** – make tea from sprouted oats and dried orange peels; drink one cup three times daily.

Pearl Barley (Job's Tears, Coix)

Nature/Taste: cool and bland

Actions: promotes diuresis, strengthens Spleen, benefits gall bladder, clears heat, detoxifies

Conditions: swelling, indigestion, diarrhea, jaundice, tumors, dysuria

Folk Remedies:
1. **For quitting coffee** – substitute roasted barley tea for coffee.

2. **Swelling** – eat pearl barley soup.
3. **Heat and damp conditions** – make a soupy porridge of mung beans and pearl barley, eat daily.
4. **Heat conditions and skin lesions** – blend barley and water, boil, and drink the liquid.
5. **Skin lesions with pus discharge** – sprinkle pearl barley powder locally.
6. **Acne** – mix pearl barley powder with aloe vera gel to make a facial mask, apply every night before bed. Leave on overnight and wash off with water on the morning.

Pearled (hulled) barley–the common variety found in supermarkets– is smaller and milder than the Chinese herb variety. Coix has a stronger taste and is more diuretic.

Quinoa

Nature/Taste: sweet, warming

Actions: tonifies Chi, strengthens Spleen, warms Yang, relieves internal coldness

Conditions: fatigue, weak digestion, obesity, low resistance to colds, loose bowels

Folk Remedies:

1. **Fatigue or obesity** – substitute quinoa for all other grains except amaranth
2. **Weak digestion and diarrhea** – toast 2 tbsp quinoa until slightly brown, steep in hot water with 3 slices of ginger and a pinch of cardamom
3. **Frequent colds** – to strengthen resistance, add 1 tbsp bee pollen, lemon juice from 1/2 of a lemon and 1 tbsp of honey into daily quinoa cereal in the morning

Rice, Brown

Nature/Taste: neutral and sweet

Actions: strengthens Spleen, nourishes Stomach, quenches thirst, relieves irritability, astringes intestines, stops diarrhea

Conditions: indigestion, diarrhea, vomiting, nausea, summer heat irritability

Folk Remedies:

1. **Bloody dysentery** – cook brown rice with a persimmon cap; eat the rice.
2. **Digestive aid** – eat fermented rice cake after each meal.
3. **Child regurgitating mother's milk** – roast rice until overdone (brownish-black), add water and cook; give the child the fluid.
4. **Diarrhea** – grind rice, charcoal and take 1-2 teaspoons each time, three times daily.
5. **Anorexia and digestive weakness** – ½ cup over-done rice (bottom of pot) mixed with cardamom, fennel and orange peel, and cooked into porridge.
6. **Difficulty urinating** – consume rice porridge continuously for one month.

Rice, Sweet

Nature/Taste: warm and sweet

Actions: warms Spleen and Stomach, tonifies Chi, astringes urine

Conditions: stomach pains due to cold, diabetes, frequent urination, obesity, anemia

Contraindications: Eating too much will cause indigestion.

Folk Remedies:

1. **Obesity** – eat sweet rice cake (mochi); a small amount is very filling.
2. **Indigestion** – make tea from malt and sweet rice sprouts.
3. **Anemia, lung tuberculosis** – cook sweet rice porridge with red dates and pearl barley and eat regularly.
4. **Spontaneous sweating** – dry-roast sweet rice and wheat bran, grind into meal; take one tablespoon three times daily.

5. **Stomach pains due to cold, diarrhea** – make sweet rice porridge with yams, lotus seeds, Chinese red dates, and a pinch of pepper.

Rice, White

Nature/Taste: slightly cool and sweet

Actions: moistens Yin, clears heat, diuretic, reduces swelling

Conditions: febrile diseases, swelling, vomiting of blood, nosebleeds, nausea

Folk Remedies:

1. **Chronic gastritis** – burn rice, powder it and take twice daily with ginger tea before meals for three consecutive days, followed by a liquid diet, avoiding cold, raw and oily foods.
2. **Vomiting due to febrile disease** – consume rice porridge.
3. **Food retention** – wash rice thoroughly, then bring rice to a boil, add aloe vera juice and drink the liquid. This will produce a loose stool and reduction of the stomach distress.

Rice Bran

Nature/Taste: neutral and sweet

Actions: dispels dampness, diuretic

Conditions: mild edema in legs and feet, high cholesterol

Folk Remedies:

1. **High cholesterol** – add rice bran to a grain dish every day for at least two months.

Rye

Nature/Taste: neutral and sweet

Actions: arrests perspiration due to weakness, strengthens stomach, fortifies Chi

Conditions: fatigue, lethargy, night or day sweats due to weakness, fetal retention (baby has died but is not yet expelled by mother)

Folk Remedies:

1. **Weakness type perspiration** – boil whole rye for 15-20 minutes, add molasses and drink the liquid.
2. **Fetal retention** – make tea from the entire rye plant and raspberry leaves, and drink as much as possible.

Spelt

Nature/Taste: sweet, slightly bitter, warm

Actions: tonifies Chi, activates blood, strengthens Spleen, clears dampness, calms spirit

Conditions: tiredness, high cholesterol, obesity, restlessness

Contraindications: gluten-sensitive patients may react to spelt. However, this is an ancient cousin of wheat that tends to create less allergic reactions than wheat.

Folk Remedies:

1. **High cholesterol** – switch to whole grains like spelt, quinoa and amaranth and take fiber supplements
2. **Obesity** – eat spelt and oat bran cereals and eliminate all refined starch from diet
3. **Restlessness** – toast 1/4 cup of spelt until slightly brown and steep in 1 cup of hot water with 1 tbsp. of chamomile for 3-5 minutes. Drink throughout the day.

Wheat

Nature/Taste: slightly cool and sweet

Actions: clears heat, quenches thirst, relieves restlessness, promotes diuresis, calms spirit, stops sweating

Conditions: dry mouth and throat, swelling, difficult urination, insomnia, irritability, restlessness, menopause, spontaneous sweating, night sweats, diarrhea, burns

Contraindications: Always use organically grown wheat. Wheat absorbs ten times more nitrates (often in chemical fertilizers) than any other grain. This could explain the high incidence of allergies to modern day wheat.

Folk Remedies:

1. **Insomnia, menopause, restlessness** – make tea from one cup wheat, 12 grams licorice, and 15 Chinese black dates. Drink one cup three times daily.
2. **Burns (Initial stages)** – make a paste of charcoaled wheat meal and sesame oil and apply locally.
3. **Swelling, difficult urination** – make tea from wheat and pearl barley.
4. **Spontaneous sweating** – make tea from wheat, crushed oyster shells and Chinese red dates.

Wheat Bran

Nature/Taste: slightly warm and sweet

Actions: calms the spirit, resolves dampness, moves stool

Conditions: agitation, swelling, high cholesterol, constipation

Contraindications: not for use in colitis; can be irritating

Folk Remedies:

1. **Restlessness and emotional instability** – make a tea of wheat bran, licorice root and Chinese jujube dates. Drink three times daily until symptoms are relieved.
2. **Constipation** – add wheat bran to diet regularly, being sure to drink plenty of water too. Psyllium seed products will also provide excellent bulk laxative action.

Wheat Germ

Nature/Taste: warm and sweet

Actions: relieves restlessness, arrests diabetes

Conditions: emotional agitation, diabetes

Contraindications: Always buy wheat germ fresh and store in the refrigerator. Due to the high oil content of wheat germ, it can become rancid if it not properly stored. Rancid oil will cause a burning sensation in the throat.

Folk Remedies:

1. **Diabetes** – make bread from 60% wheat germ and 40% whole-wheat flour with an egg added in. Ideally, consume up to 1½ pounds of wheat germ per day.

Beans and Peas (Legumes)

Azuki Bean (Aduki, Red)

Nature/Taste: neutral, sweet and sour

Actions: strengthens Spleen, benefits diabetes, counteracts toxins, reduces dampness, benefits Kidney

Conditions: mumps, diabetes, leukorrhea, excessive thirst, hunger, excretion of fluids, edema

Folk Remedies:
1. **Diabetes** – after soaking red beans, boil two hours; drink the liquid three times daily.
2. **Mumps** – mash sprouted red beans and apply, either alone or mixed with dandelion.

Black Bean

Nature/Taste: warm and sweet

Actions: tonifies Kidney, nourishes the Yin, strengthens and nourishes blood, brightens eyes, promotes urination

Conditions: lower back pain, knee pain, infertility, seminal emissions, blurry vision, ear problems, difficult urination

Folk Remedies:
1. **Beriberi** – cook black beans with carp.
2. **Spontaneous menopausal sweating** – make boiled black bean juice.
3. **Low back pain, weak knees, frequent urination, and other Kidney weakness symptoms** – slowly cook (for about 2 -3 hours) ½ cup black beans, ½ cup water, and ¾ cup rice wine. This is a good winter tonic.
4. **Kidney stones** – add kombu seaweed to the above winter tonic.
5. **Bedwetting** – include black beans in the diet regularly.

Garbanzo Bean (Chickpea)

Nature/Taste: sweet, slightly warm

Actions: strengthens Spleen, tonifies Chi, calms spirit, clears dampness, promotes bowel movement

Conditions: low energy, anxiety, restlessness, constipation, lack of concentration

Folk Remedies:

1. **Low energy** – eat hummus made from garbonzos as a snack between meals. You can use it as a dip for vegetable sticks like carrots, celery and jicama sticks instead of crackers or pita bread.
2. **Anxiety and restlessness** – make hummus with garbonzos as well as herbs like parsley, basil and chives
3. **Constipation** – regularly eat garbonzo bean soup cooked with beets, turnip, and squashes

Kidney Bean

Nature/Taste: neutral and sweet

Actions: strengthens digestion, promotes elimination, diuretic

Conditions: swelling, difficulty urinating, diarrhea

Folk Remedies:

1. **Swelling due to nephritis** – make a strong soup with ½ cup beans to five cups of water, cooked down to one cup.
2. **Chronic diarrhea** – roast kidney beans, then cook with rice water (the soaking water) to make a tea.

Lentil

Nature/Taste: slightly warm and sweet

Actions: harmonizes digestion, strengthens stomach, descends rebellious Chi, clears summer heat

Conditions: cholera, vomiting, diarrhea, dysentery

Folk Remedies:
1. **Summer diarrhea, dysentery** – grind lentils into meal and mix with rice porridge and eat.
2. **Heatstroke with fever, restlessness, and difficult urination** – eat cool lentil soup.

Lima Bean

Nature/Taste: sweet, cool

Actions: tonifies Chi, nourishes blood, clears heat, resolves dampness, promotes bowel movement, strengthens Lung, calms spirit

Conditions: tiredness, sinus allergies, rashes, hives, high cholesterol, constipation, anxiety, insomnia, anemia

Folk Remedies:
1. **Tiredness and anemia** – puree lima beans with roasted garlic and fresh basil and eat in between meals.
2. **Insomnia** – eat soup for dinner made from lima beans with other calming foods like turkey and sage.
3. **Allergic reaction to sulfites** – make broth from boiling equal portions of lima and mung beans. Drink 3 cups daily.

Mung Bean

Nature/Taste: very cool and sweet

Actions: clears heat, detoxifies, quenches thirst, promotes urination, reduces swelling, aids edema in the lower limbs, counteracts toxins

Conditions: edema, conjunctivitis, diabetes, dysentery, summer heat conditions, heatstroke, dehydration, food poisoning from spoiled food, carbuncles

Contraindications: not for cold conditions. Females should avoid mung beans if trying to get pregnant.

Folk Remedies:

1. **Dysentery** – take five parts mung beans to one part black pepper; grind to a powder and take one tablespoon three times daily. Usually one will notice results in 6 -12 hours. The black pepper acts as an antibacterial agent.
2. **Breast abscess and boils** – take two tablespoons mung bean powder in warm water twice daily.
3. **Hives and bad skin lesions** – make mung bean juice in a blender and drink raw.
4. **Summer heat conditions** – make soup from mung beans, barley, and rice.

Sweet and cold, mung bean sprouts clear heat and toxins as well as generate fluids.

Navy Bean

Nature/Taste: Sweet, warm

Actions: tonifies Chi, nourishes blood, activates blood, removes stagnation, improves memory, calms spirit

Conditions: anemia, memory decline, high cholesterol, blood sugar imbalance, fatigue

Contraindication: gout

Folk Remedies:

1. **Memory decline** – make a brain tonic bean soup by cooking equal portions of navy beans, black beans and kidney beans and seasoned with rosemary, thyme and tumeric. Eat a bowl daily.
2. **Diabetes** – incorporate navy beans and other beans into diet to help balance the blood sugar level.
3. **Anemia** – cooked up a hearty white chili with navy beans, ground chicken, and chopped parsley. Eat daily.

Pea

Nature/Taste: neutral and sweet

Actions: strengthens digestion, strengthens Spleen and Stomach, promotes urination, lubricates intestines

Conditions: indigestion, edema, constipation

Folk Remedies:

1. **Edema** – roast peas until dry, powder and take with warm water.
2. **Indigestion** – blend peas into a juice and take with meals.

Pinto Bean

Nature/Taste: sweet, warm

Actions: tonifies Chi, nourishes blood, clears heat, resolves dampness, calms spirit

Conditions: fatigue, anemia, edema, sulfite allergies, high cholesterol, insomnia, anxiety

Folk Remedies:

1. **High cholesterol** – incorporate pinto beans and other beans into your regular diet that are high in fiber and contain rich folate that lowers cholesterol
2. **Edema and swelling** – make broth from boiling pinto beans with cabbage for 1/2 hour, strain and drink 1 cup of broth, 3 times a day until swelling improves. Season with herbs and spices, but avoid adding salt to the broth.
3. **Anxiety** – eat hummus made from pinto beans, lima beans and garbonzos beans reguarly

Soybean

Nature/Taste: cool and sweet

Actions: clears heat, detoxifies, eases urination, lubricates lungs and intestines, provides an excellent protein source

Conditions: Lung and Stomach heat, dry skin, intense appetite, stomach or mouth ulcers, swollen gums, diarrhea, constipation, general heat problems

Contraindications: Do not eat soybeans raw; they cannot be digested.

Folk Remedies:
1. **Heat conditions** – drink soymilk or eat tofu. Soymilk is easily made by blending soaked soybeans with a larger volume of water; strain off the milk and bring to a boil for about twenty minutes; sweeten to taste. To make tofu, curdle the soymilk with calcium sulfate, nigari, or lemon juice; strain and press the solids into a block.
2. **Diarrhea** – charcoal soybeans and grind to a powder; take one teaspoon three times daily.
3. **Habitual constipation** – boil tea from soybeans and drink four times daily.

Tofu, Soybean Curd

Nature/Taste: cool and sweet

Actions: clears heat, lubricates dryness, promotes body fluids, detoxifies, strengthens Spleen and Stomach

Conditions: chronic dysentery, malaria, lung tuberculosis, anemia, leukorrhea, irregular menstruation

Folk Remedies:
1. **Chronic dysentery** – stir-fry tofu with vinegar.
2. **Malaria** – stir-fry tofu with vinegar; take three hours prior to the onset of symptoms.
3. **Lung tuberculosis** – combine tofu and the herb, Alismatis rhizome (water plantain tuber); boil, and eat the tofu. Take daily for two months.
4. **Anemia** – take frozen tofu that has been thawed, mix with egg white, until the egg white has soaked into the tofu; cook and eat daily for one month.

5. **Leukorrhea** – steam tofu and brown sugar.
6. **Irregular menstruation due to coldness** – stew together tofu, lamb, and ginger.

To reduce the cool nature of tofu, press out the extra water, marinate with ginger and garlic, then bake. This would be more suitable for conditions of cold or dampness. Baked tofu is widely available in Asian and health food markets.

Nuts and Seeds

Almond
Nature/Taste: neutral and sweet

Actions: ventilates Lungs, relieves cough and asthma, transforms phlegm, lubricates intestines

Conditions: lung conditions, asthma, constipation, cough

Folk Remedies:
1. **Cough and asthma** – grind almonds to a fine meal, add fructose; dissolve two tablespoons in water.

Cashews
Nature/Taste: sweet, warm

Actions: tonifies Kidney, strengthens bones, nourishes blood, boosts Chi, moistens Yin, promotes bowel movement

Conditions: lower back pain, osteopenia, frequent urination, dizziness, fatigue, low libido, infertility, constipation

Contraindications: dampness, diarrhea

Folk Remedies:
1. **Lower back pain** – make curry cashews by dry roasting cashews in a pan and sprinkle with curry powder for a couple of minutes on high flame. Remove promptly and do not burn the cashews. Eat a handful a day.
2. **Infertility or low libido** – make a libido and fertility enhancing trail mix consisting of equal parts of dried cranberry, walnut, sesame seeds, longan fruit, and cashews.
3. **Constipation** – ground cashews into powder. Mix 1 tsp. cashew powder and 1 tbsp. honey into a cup of hot water and drink on empty stomach upon waking each morning.

Chestnut
Nature/Taste: warm, sweet and salty

Actions: tonifies Kidney, strengthens digestion, fortifies the Chi, arrests cough

Conditions: weak Kidney Chi, back pain, weak lower extremities, frequent urination, nausea, burping, hiccups, chronic bronchitis, cough, asthma, diarrhea

Folk Remedies:

1. **Diarrhea** – grind chestnuts to flour and boil for 10-15 minutes, then consume the porridge.
2. **Chronic cough, bronchitis** – eat steamed chestnuts and drink chestnut leaf tea.
3. **Nausea, hiccups, gastritis** – charcoal and powder the membrane (not the shell) of the chestnut and cook about 1½ -3 grams into rice porridge.
4. **Kidney weakness, back or leg pain, frequent urination** – eat two raw chestnuts daily, one in the morning and one at night; chew thoroughly.
5. **Splinters, traumas, sores** – mash raw chestnuts and apply to the affected area to draw out a splinter or pus, reduce pain and stop bleeding.

Filbert, Hazelnut

Nature/Taste: neutral and sweet

Actions: fortifies Chi, strengthens digestion

Conditions: diarrhea, lack of appetite

Folk Remedies:

1. **Diarrhea** – roast filberts and grind into meal; take one teaspoon twice daily with jujube date tea.
2. **Lack of appetite** – grind raw filberts into a meal; take one teaspoon twice daily with tea made from citrus peel.

Lotus Seed

Nature/Taste: neutral and sweet

Actions: strengthens Kidney, astringent, nutritive tonic

Conditions: Kidney weakness, frequent urination, involuntary seminal emission, diarrhea

Folk Remedies:
1. **Nutritive tonic** – a delicious winter tonic soup can be made by boiling together lotus seeds, azuki (red) beans, and pearl barley; add a dash of honey before serving.
2. **Frequent urination, involuntary seminal emission, diarrhea** – cook lotus seeds and cubes of sweet potato in a rice porridge.

Peanut

Nature/Taste: neutral and sweet

Actions: improves appetite, strengthens Spleen, regulates blood, lubricates lungs, promotes diuresis, aids in lactation

Conditions: edema, difficult lactation, blood in urine, insomnia, lack of appetite

Folk Remedies:
1. **Edema** – drink peanut tea for seven consecutive days.
2. **Lack of milk** – steam peanuts, mash, and add to soupy rice.
3. **Chronic cough** – combine peanuts, jujube dates, and honey; make tea and drink twice daily.
4. **Chronic nephritis** – combine peanuts and red dates; make tea and eat the solids. Take for one week.
5. **Insomnia** – boil peanut tea; drink in the evening.
6. **Hypertension** – take peanut shells and boil tea or grind into powder and take with warm water; drink three times daily for at least twenty days.

Pecan

Nature/Taste: sweet, slightly warm

Actions: tonifies Chi, strengthens Lung, stops cough, strengthens Kidney, promotes bowel movement

Conditions: fatigue, chronic cough, lower back pain, low libido, erectile dysfunction, frequent urination, constipation

Contraindications: dampness, diarrhea

Folk Remedies:

1. **Chronic cough** – ground pecan into powder. Mix 1 tbsp. each of pecan powder, apricot seed/kernel powder and honey into 1 cup of hot water. Drink 2-3 cups daily.
2. **Lower back pain** – soak pecan in sherry or port for one week or more. Eat a small handful daily.
3. **Erectile dysfunction or low libido** – make a libido- and fertility-enhancing trail mix consisting of equal parts of goji berry, pecan, raisin, and pistachios. Eat a small handful each day.

Pine Nut

Nature/Taste: warm and sweet

Actions: lubricates lungs, relieves cough, lubricates intestines, promotes production of body fluids

Conditions: dry cough, constipation

Contraindications: not to be used with diarrhea, involuntary seminal emission, or any mucous conditions.

Folk Remedies:

1. **Dry cough** – grind pine nuts and walnuts, add honey and slowly cook over low flame until thick; take two teaspoons with warm water.
2. **Constipation** – eat pine nuts with rice porridge.

Pumpkin Seed

Nature/Taste: cold and sweet

Actions: anti-parasitic, diuretic

Conditions: intestinal worms and parasites, swelling, diabetes, prostate problems

Folk Remedies:

1. **Intestinal worms** – roast and powder pumpkin seeds, then mix with honey and take twice daily. Or eat a large handful of pumpkin seeds 2-3 times a day.

2. **Swelling after pregnancy, diabetes** – make a tea from roasted pumpkin seeds.
3. **Prostate problems** – eat a large handful of pumpkin seeds twice daily.

Sesame Seed, Brown

Nature/Taste: slightly warm and sweet

Actions: nourishes Liver and Kidney, lubricates intestines, blackens gray hair, overall body tonic, benefits skin

Conditions: backache, weakness, premature graying, ringing in the ears, blurry vision, dizziness, constipation, dry cough, blood in the urine, tonic for older people, weak knees

Contraindications: Always grind seeds because the tough cell wall makes whole seeds indigestible.

Folk Remedies:

1. **Weakness conditions, constipation** – grind sesame seeds to a meal, mix with honey to make a paste; take two teaspoons twice daily.
2. **Dry cough and asthma** – roast sesame seeds, grind to a meal and add ginger juice and honey. Take one teaspoon three times daily.

Sesame Seed, Black

Nature/Taste: neutral and sweet

Actions: tonifies Liver and Kidney, harmonizes the blood, lubricates intestines, restores hair color, nourishes Yin, promotes lactation

Conditions: chronic constipation, premature balding or graying, chronic arthritis, joint inflammation, cough

Folk Remedies:

1. **Chronic constipation** – grind into a meal and mix with honey and form small chewable balls, about 6 grams each. Take one ball three times daily with rice wine.

2. **Premature balding or graying** – grind both black sesames and black beans to a meal; cook with rice milk. Take once daily for at least three months.
3. **Chronic cough, asthma** – grind equal parts black sesame seeds and apricot kernels; take one teaspoon with warm water three times daily.

Sunflower Seed

Nature/Taste: neutral and sweet

Actions: subdues Liver, lowers blood pressure, relieves dysentery, resolves pus, moistens intestines

Conditions: headache, dizziness, liver-fire rising, bloody dysentery, intestinal worms

Folk Remedies:
1. **Headache or dizziness** – grind the seeds and take with honey and warm water before bed.
2. **Hypertension** – take sunflower seed meal with celery juice.
3. **Bloody dysentery** – cook the seeds with water of one hour, add honey; drink the liquid and eat the seeds.

Walnut

Nature/Taste: slightly warm and sweet

Actions: tonifies Kidney, strengthens back, astringes Lung, relieves asthma, lubricates intestines, aids erratic or rebellious Chi, reduces cholesterol

Conditions: Kidney deficiency, impotency, sexual dysfunctions, infertility, frequent urination, back and leg pain, stones in the urinary tract, cough, constipation, neurasthenia

Folk Remedies:
1. **Impotence and Kidney weakness** – eat twenty walnuts a day for one month.

2. **Back pain and cold type arthritis** – take walnut meal with warm wine (preferably red wine).
3. **Kidney stones** – take 120 grams walnuts, grind to a meal and add 120 grams brown sugar; roast with sesame oil. Take ¼ of the mixture four times a day.
4. **Neurasthenia** – take equal portions of walnuts, sesame seeds, and dried mulberries, mash together to a paste; roll into small pills and take three pills three times a day.
5. **Cough, constipation** – grind walnuts into meal and mix with honey. Take two tablespoons daily with warm water.

Winter Melon Seed

Nature/Taste: cool and bland

Actions: promotes diuresis, resolves mucus, stops cough, clears heat, detoxifies

Conditions: coughing of blood, constipation, intestinal abscess, edema, leukorrhea

Folk Remedies:

1. **Coughing of blood, constipation, and intestinal abscess** – make tea from the seeds.
2. **Edema and leukorrhea** – grind seeds into meal and take one teaspoon with warm water three times daily.
3. **Edema in the summer** – cook soup with winter melon peel (purchased dry), winter melon seed, mung beans and pearl barley.
4. **Coughing blood** – make tea from winter melon seed, pearl barley and fresh lotus root.

Meat, Fish, Poultry and Animal Products

Meat, fish, poultry and eggs should always be properly cooked and never eaten raw. Seek producers that treat animals humanely and do not use drugs.

Eating fish that comes from around the world helps avoid mercury exposure. Try not to eat fish from the same region in the same week, as eating fish from a variety of locations diminishes your risk of repeated exposure to the same toxins. The larger the fish, the more mercury accumulates. For example, tuna, swordfish and shark have been found to have larger amounts of mercury. Fresh sardines, which are small, have very little mercury. Pregnant women should eat no more than 2-3 servings of fish per week.

For complete lists of safe fish to eat, visit: www.seafoodwatch.org.

Beef

Nature/Taste: warm and sweet

Actions: tonifies Chi and blood, strengthens Spleen and Stomach, dispels dampness, relieves edema, strengthens bones and tendons

Conditions: edema, abdominal distention and fullness, weak back and knees, deficient Stomach and Spleen

Contraindications: not to be used with any type of skin lesions, hepatitis, or any kind of kidney inflammation.

Folk Remedies:

1. **Deficiencies of blood, Chi, Spleen** – take cooked ground beef and soak it in hot water for 10 minutes; drink the juice.
2. **Edema or chronic diarrhea** – stew beef in water for two hours; drink the liquid.

Chicken

Nature/Taste: warm and sweet

Actions: tonifies Chi, nourishes blood, aids Kidney deficiency, benefits Spleen and Stomach

Conditions: postpartum weakness, weakness in old people, cold-type arthritis, weakness after illness or blood loss

Contraindications: Do not eat chickens that are force fed chemical pellets and injected with steroids and antibiotics. These chickens can cause a variety of health problems, including sterility, early female puberty, disharmony in the menstrual cycle, male impotence, to name a few. Also, chicken is not to be consumed by those with heat type cancers such as leukemia, or when there are heat symptoms such as red tongue, fever, and extreme thirst.

Folk Remedies:

1. **Weakness or anemia** – cook one chicken with 30 grams dang gui (Angelica sinensis), and 6½ cups water. Simmer together for one hour. The darker meat birds such as the Chinese black chicken are the most tonifying.

Turkey is also warm but not as tonifying as chicken.

Chicken Egg

Nature/Taste: cool and sweet

Actions: nourishes Yin, tonifies blood, stabilizes hyperactive fetus, lubricates dryness

Conditions: dry cough, hoarse voice, dysentery, blood and Yin deficiency, hyperactive fetus

Contraindications: Eating too many eggs is not healthy. In general, do not eat fried or raw eggs.

Folk Remedies:

1. **Yin and blood deficiency** – steam the eggs and eat.
2. **Postpartum** – eat eggs with green onions.
3. **Pain of dysentery** – cook eggs with rice vinegar.
4. **Hyperactive fetus** – eat a hard boiled egg daily.

Duck

Nature/Taste: sweet, salty, neutral

Actions: tonifies Chi, nourishes Yin, moistens dryness, nourishes Kidney and Lung, relieves edema

Conditions: dry cough, postpartum weakness, fatigue, swelling due to kidney weakness

Contraindications: duck tends to be greasy and hard on people with weak digestion

Folk Remedies:

1. **Postpartum fatigue and weakness** – cook duck with ginger, scallions and black beans
2. **Weak lungs with dry cough** – make duck soup with apricot seed/kernel, lily bulbs and Asian pears
3. **Kidney weakness with edema** – make salad with shredded duck breast meat, cucumber, celery and sweet onions

Fish

Nature/Taste: warm* and sweet

Actions: strengthens Spleen, tonifies Chi, removes dampness, regulates blood, aids diarrhea from Spleen weakness

Conditions: low energy states, hemorrhoids, postpartum excessive bleeding, itching or exuding damp type skin lesions

Contraindications: Do not eat fish raw as it is often loaded with parasites. Always cook fish with garlic, ginger or onion to neutralize potential toxins.

Folk Remedies:

1. **Kidney deficiency and back pain** – cook fish with chicken.

* *Ocean fish are energetically cooler than freshwater fish. Many ocean fish are considered neutral. Clams and crabs are cool, oysters are neutral, and shrimp is warm. Shellfish can cause rashes and other allergic reactions.*

Goat's Milk

Nature/Taste: sweet, salty, warm

Actions: tonifies Chi, nourishes blood, strengthens Kidney and builds strong bones, moistens dryness, calms spirit

Conditions: fatigue, diabetes, metabolic syndrome, weak bone health, anemia, dry skin and hair, insomnia, nervousness

Contraindications: fevers

Folk Remedies:

1. **Metabolic syndrome or blood sugar imbalance** – substitute goat milk and goat yogurt for cow milk and ice cream.
2. **Osteopenia or osteoporosis** – make bone-building hummus with black beans and goat milk yogurt. Eat as a snack in between meals regularly.
3. **Dry skin and hair** – once a week, condition hair with goat milk by rubbing a cup of goat milk into hair and body in the shower and let it remain for 10 minutes before washing off.

Lamb

Nature/Taste: hot and sweet

Actions: tonifies weakness, dispels cold, strengthens and nourishes Chi and blood, promotes appetite, aids lactation

Conditions: Kidney deficiency causing back pain, impotence, cold conditions, deficiency conditions, postpartum blood loss, lack of milk, leukorrhea

Contraindications: Lamb is generally not consumed in summer because of its hot nature. It is not to be consumed in conditions of edema, malaria, common cold, toothache and any type of heat conditions.

Folk Remedies:

1. **Anemia, weakness, blood deficiency** – cook lamb with ginger and dang gui (Angelica sinensis). In general, meats are traditionally prepared with such herbs as dang gui, jujube date, astragalus, ginger, scallions, or ginseng for problems of weakness and coldness.

Milk and Milk Products

Nature/Taste: neutral and sweet

Actions: strengthens weakness, nourishes Chi and blood, lubricates dryness

Conditions: nutritional deficiency, weakness, malnutrition, anemia, constipation, dryness

Contraindications: not to be used with damp or cold conditions, or in cases of diarrhea. In general not to be used by adults or those who are healthy as dairy products can cause mucus and other disorders. As an occasional food used moderately, dairy products should not cause a problem; however, they are not to be used daily. Allergy is common with this food since many adults lose the ability to digest milk sugar after infancy. Allergic reactions usually include diarrhea and bloating.

Folk Remedies:

1. **Weakness, malnutrition** – drink a glass of warm milk.

Pork

Nature/Taste: slightly cold and sweet

Actions: moistens and nourishes organs, tonifies Chi, strengthens digestion

Conditions: internal dryness, constipation, dry cough, emaciation

Contraindications: not to be taken by overweight people, those with deficient Spleen and Stomach, hypertension, stroke victims, or those with diarrhea.

Folk Remedies:

1. **Constipation, dry cough** – make soup with pork, carrots and lily bulbs.
2. **Weakness, emaciation** – cook pork in a rice porridge.

Quail Egg

Nature/Taste: sweet, salty, warm

Actions: tonifies Chi, restores Jing, warms Yang, resolves dampness, improves vision, activates blood and removes stagnation

Conditions: fatigue, memory decline, loss of concentration, infertility, cataract, age-related macular degeneration, blood clots, arthritic inflammation

Contraindications: people with egg allergies

Folk Remedies:

1. **Infertility or inadequate sperm** – 3 fresh quail eggs in a shot glass mixed with 1 oz. of clear alcohol like gin or vodka. Drink before bedtime daily for 1 month. (Note: alcohol is necessary to prevent salmonella. If alcohol is not preferred, eat the eggs cooked.)
2. **Vision decline** – scramble quail eggs with spinach and carrots for breakfast daily
3. **Memory and focus issues** – eat hardboiled quail eggs regularly

Miscellaneous Foods, Herbs and Beverages

Anise

Nature/Taste: warm and pungent

Actions: strengthens stomach, regulates Chi flow, harmonizes Stomach, stops vomiting

Conditions: hernia, beriberi, abdominal pain, distention and gas, back pain and coldness, cold stomach

Contraindications: not to be used in any type of heat conditions.

Folk Remedies:

1. **Stomach pain due to coldness** – make anise tea and add some wine.
2. **Hernia** – charcoal anise and grind to powder; add brown sugar and take with rice wine.

Barley Malt Syrup

Nature/Taste: neutral and sweet

Actions: promotes digestion, relieves food stagnation, strengthens stomach, stops lactation

Conditions: food retention caused by wheat products, epigastric fullness and distention, belching, constipation, undesirable lactation

Folk Remedies:

1. **Food retention and stopping lactation** – drink barley malt in warm water until condition resolves.

Rice malt syrup is neutral and sweet and has properties similar to barley malt, except that rice malt is preferred for food stagnation caused by rice products.

Basil

Nature/Taste: warm and pungent

Actions: induces sweating, harmonizes Stomach, antidote for seafood poisoning

Conditions: wind-cold, vomiting, diarrhea, seafood poisoning

Folk Remedies:

1. **Common cold** – boil tea from basil, ginger, and green onions.
2. **Diarrhea, vomiting, seafood poisoning** – boil basil tea.

Black Fungus (Wood Ears)

Nature/Taste: neutral and sweet, slightly toxic when raw

Actions: nourishes Stomach, calms spirit, lubricates dryness, promotes blood flow, removes stagnation

Conditions: blood stagnation such as tumor, especially uterine, abnormal uterine bleeding, bloody stools, hemorrhoids, constipation, hypertension

Contraindications: not to be used by pregnant women.

Folk Remedies:

1. **Hypertension, bloody stools, and hemorrhoids** – add honey to some black fungus and dried persimmon, cook, and eat once a day.
2. **Abnormal bleeding, anemia** – boil tea from black fungus and Chinese dates.
3. **Dysentery** – take 10 grams fresh black fungus with warm water twice daily.
4. **Tumors of the viscera and female organs** – make tea from black fungus and peach kernel, and drink.

Black Pepper

Nature/Taste: hot and pungent

Actions: warms digestion, dispels internal cold, antidote to food poisoning

Conditions: stomachache due to cold, diarrhea, food poisoning

Folk Remedies:
1. **Food poisoning** – mix one teaspoon black pepper with rice porridge and grated ginger and drink as much as possible.

Brown Sugar, Turbinado

Nature/Taste: warm and sweet

Actions: strengthens digestion, lubricates lungs, stops cough, warms up the body

Conditions: dry cough, poor digestion, coldness

Contraindications: not to be consumed in excess, can lead to mucus and dampness in the body.

Folk Remedies:
1. **Stomach pains, ulcer pains** – mix a spoonful of brown sugar into warm water and drink to arrest pain.
2. **Dry cough, sore throat** – grate carrots and mix with brown sugar. Refrigerate overnight, then consume the next day.

White sugar is sweet and cold; it lubricates the lungs and treats dry cough; it can be used externally to promote the healing of bed sores, ulcerations and burns. Apply sugar to the lesion and re-handage every 3-5 days. The same contraindications for brown sugar apply to white sugar.

Cardamom Seed

Nature/Taste: warm and pungent

Actions: warms digestion, resolves dampness, invigorates the flow of Chi, stops vomiting

Conditions: dampness, diarrhea, nausea, vomiting, stomach ulcers, abdominal distention and fullness

Folk Remedies:
1. **Stomach and duodenal ulcers** – drink cardamom and fresh ginger root tea on an empty stomach every morning.

2. **Abdominal pain and distention** – make tea from cardamom, cloves and orange peel. Drink three times daily.
3. **Nausea and diarrhea** – stir one teaspoon cardamom powder into one cup warm water and drink three times daily.

Carob Pod

Nature/Taste: warm and sweet

Actions: soothes and calms the spirit

Conditions: used as an alternative to chocolate, and for caffeine addiction

Contraindications: Eating carob to excess will cause agitation.

Folk Remedies:

1. **Chocolate substitute** – use powdered carob pods.

Cinnamon

Nature/Taste: hot, pungent and sweet

Actions: strengthens stomach, warms any coldness in the body, stops pain

Conditions: common cold, abdominal pain due to cold stagnation, lack of appetite due to cold stomach, low back pain

Contraindications: not to be used in pregnancy.

Folk Remedies:

1. **Postpartum abdominal pain** – boil tea with cinnamon and brown sugar.
2. **Premenstrual syndrome, including lower abdominal pain and bloating prior to menstruation** – make tea from cinnamon and hawthorn berries.
3. **Gas pain in stomach area** – take ½ teaspoon cinnamon powder with lukewarm water, twice daily.

Cloves

Nature/Taste: warm and pungent

Actions: warms the middle of the body, dispels internal cold, reverses rebellious Chi, warms Kidney, stops pain

Conditions: stomachache due to cold, vomiting, nausea, belching, hiccupping, toothache

Folk Remedies:

1. **Vomiting, nausea, belching** – drink one teaspoon clove powder in warm water.
2. **Toothache** – place clove above or below the affected tooth on the gum until pain is relieved.

Coffee

Nature/Taste: warm, sweet and bitter

Actions: stimulating, diuretic, promotes elimination

Conditions: mild swelling, constipation, hypersomnia, lethargy, mental cloudiness, conditions that require stimulation

Contraindications: This beverage is a very addictive substance. Avoid in high blood pressure, insomnia, nervousness, and stomach ulcers or acidity. Coffee is easier on the stomach if taken with milk or soymilk. Always exercise moderation in its use. Avoid during pregnancy.

Fennel

Nature/Taste: warm and pungent

Actions: unblocks and regulates Chi, strengthens stomach, dispels cold, stops pain, stimulates peristalsis

Conditions: stomachache, hernia, abdominal discomfort, coldness is the stomach, colic in babies

Folk Remedies:

1. **Hernia** – boil tea from fennel seeds, black pepper, cinnamon, and orange peel. Externally apply warming liniment along with a heating pad.

Ginger Root [Fresh]

Nature/Taste: warm and pungent

Actions: promotes sweating, anti-toxin, antidote for seafood poisoning, benefits Lung and Stomach, expels pathogens

Conditions: common cold, cough due to coldness (clear or white mucus), nausea, vomiting, diarrhea, cold-type arthritis

Folk Remedies:

1. **Colds, cough, vomiting** – drink ginger tea.
2. **Diarrhea** – apply ginger plaster to the belly.
3. **Baldness** – rub fresh ginger on the scalp.
4. **Arthritis** – rub fresh ginger on painful areas and drink tea (not for heat-type arthritis).
5. **Nausea** – squeeze ginger juice into some water and sip slowly until nausea is reduced.

Dried ginger is hot and pungent and should be used to dispel coldness. For stomach or abdominal pain, drink tea made from dried ginger and cloves.

Honey

Nature/Taste: neutral, unless heated, then it is warm and sweet

Actions: nourishes Yin, lubricates dryness, tonifies weakness, harmonizes, antidote to drugs, strengthens Spleen

Conditions: diabetes (small amounts), constipation, ulcers, dry cough, hoarse voice, burns, cold sores

Contraindications: not to be used in diarrhea or conditions of dampness or phlegm.

Folk Remedies:

1. **Ulcers** – mix honey and ginger juice and take on an empty stomach every morning.
2. **Burns** – apply locally.
3. **Cough, constipation, and hoarseness** – mix honey with water and/or almonds.

Avoid heating honey unless a warming nature is desired; heating lowers the nourishing and beneficial effects. The darker honeys are more tonifying and tend to sink to the lower parts of the body. The lighter honeys are better for upper body problems.

Molasses

Nature/Taste: warm and sweet

Actions: tonifies Chi, strengthens Spleen, lubricates lungs, stops cough

Conditions: stomach and abdominal pain, Chi deficiency, cough

Folk Remedies:

1. **Stomach or duodenal ulcers** – take two teaspoons of molasses in lukewarm water to stop pain.
2. **Cough** – dice carrots, mix with molasses and leave it overnight; take two teaspoons three times daily.
3. **Bedwetting** – boil cinnamon and licorice tea, adding two teaspoons of molasses.

Olive

Nature/Taste: neutral, sweet, sour and astringent

Actions: clears heat, detoxifies, promotes production of body fluids, quenches thirst, clears lungs, benefits the throat

Conditions: whooping cough, dysentery, sore throat, dehydration, laryngitis, thirst

Folk Remedies:

1. **Cough and dry conditions** – eat olives regularly.
2. **Sore, dry throat and laryngitis** – take fifty black, pitted olives with 3-4 cups of honey; heat over a low flame. Take 2-3 tablespoons three times daily, swallowing slowly.

Rice Vinegar

Nature/Taste: warm and sour

Actions: detoxifies, invigorates blood circulation, inhibits growth of bacteria, astringent, closes pores

Conditions: preventative for common colds, prevents invasion from external pathogens, malaria, acute arthritis, vomiting, nausea, intestinal worms, hypertension, burns, fungus infestation, bones caught in the throat, gum disease, hives, hepatitis, lung tuberculosis, lung abscess, bronchitis

Contraindications: not to be used at the onset of a cold as it will trap pathogens inside of the body.

Folk Remedies:

1. **Malaria** – mix 2-3 tablespoons of rice vinegar with two teaspoons baking soda; take two hours before the episodic attacks of chills and fever.
2. **Acute arthritis** – boil two cups rice vinegar down to one cup; add green onions and boil another five minutes. Soak gauze pad and apply to sore area twice daily until condition improves.
3. **Nausea and vomiting** – mix equal parts rice vinegar and water and drink.
4. **Intestinal worms** – take rice vinegar with water on an empty stomach.
5. **Hypertension** – soak peanuts in vinegar; eat twenty peanuts every morning.
6. **Burns** – apply undiluted.
7. **Fish bones in the throat** – slowly drink one cup vinegar, and then eat a hard bread crust.
8. **Gum disease** – rinse mouth often with undiluted vinegar.
9. **Hives** – make ginger tea, add rice vinegar and brown sugar; drink twice daily.
10. **Hepatitis** – soak apple-pear in vinegar; eat daily.
11. **Lung tuberculosis** – soak garlic in rice vinegar for 2-7 days; take one clove twice daily.

12. **Lung abscess** – boil garlic in vinegar; eat 1-2 cloves daily.
13. **Bronchitis** – combine ten mashed garlic cloves, one cup vinegar, and two teaspoons brown sugar; take two tea spoons three times daily.

Salt

Nature/Taste: cold, salty and slightly sweet

Actions: harmonizes and promotes digestion, strengthens Kidney (in small amounts), fortifies bones, tendons and teeth, brightens eyes, detoxifies, used as a natural preservative

Conditions: food poisoning, Kidney weakness from lack of sodium in the diet, sore throat

Folk Remedies:
1. **Food poisoning** – for immediate relief, roast salt and take with warm water which will cause vomiting to relieve condition.
2. **Itchy, inflamed skin** – wash area with salt water or apply salt.
3. **Sore throat** – gargle with warm salt water several times a day.

Spirulina/Chlorella

Nature/Taste: salty, cool

Actions: tonifies Chi, nourishes Yin and blood, strengthens Kidney, clears heat toxins from Liver

Conditions: low energy, anemia, kidney weakness, lower back pain, weak knees, night sweat, irritability, agitation, hepatitis, liver toxicity, indigestion

Folk Remedies:
1. **Low energy and anemia** – make a shake from 1 tbsp spirulina or chlorella with raspberry, banana and goat yogurt. Drink daily

2. **Liver toxicity** – make vegetable juice from chard, kale, spinach, beet and carrot greens, carrot, apple and 1 tbsp of spirulina or chlorella. Consume 1-2 glasses daily

3. **Kidney and low back or knee weakness** – eat a rich breakfast cereal by cooking together any of the following: black beans, kidney beans, adzuki beans, chestnuts, walnuts, sesame seeds, amaranth, quinoa, millet. Sprinkle 1 tbsp. spirulina or chlorella and 1 tbsp. flax seed meal to a bowl of this cereal daily.

Tea

Nature/Taste: cool, bitter and sweet

Actions: clears the head, refreshes the mind, relieves thirst and restlessness, resolves phlegm, diuretic, promotes digestion, detoxifies, reduces cholesterol

Conditions: headaches, blurry vision, thirst, restlessness, foggy head, hypersomnia, food retention, dysentery, difficulty urinating, overweight

Contraindications: Avoid or use minimally with insomnia. Due to tannin, better not to drink tea on an empty stomach.

Folk Remedies:

1. **For the conditions listed above** – prepare tea leaves (preferably green tea) and drink as needed.

White Fungus (Silver Ears)

Nature/Taste: neutral and sweet

Actions: clears Lung heat, strengthens Spleen and Stomach, promotes body fluids, tonifies Chi, invigorates blood, lubricates intestines, relieves alcohol intoxication, nourishes Yin

Conditions: cough, dry lungs, bloody sputum, irregular menstruation, arteriosclerosis, hypertension, alcohol intoxication, blood stagnation, constipation

Folk Remedies:

1. **Lung problems, constipation, bloody sputum** – soak white fungus for twelve hours, add honey, and steam. Drink the liquid on an empty stomach. This is known as *silver ears soup*.
2. **Arteriosclerosis, hypertension, eye hemorrhage** – drink silver ears soup before bedtime.
3. **Weakness after long illness or loss of blood** – slowly stew white fungus, ten Chinese dates, and either pork or chicken.

Wine

Nature/Taste: warm, pungent and sweet

Actions: promotes circulation, enhances the effect of circulatory herbs, temporarily stops pain

Conditions: arthritis, traumas, bruises, painful conditions

Contraindications: wine can be a very addictive substance. In case of allergy to alcohol, avoid it completely. Wine is not recommended for heat conditions. Avoid during pregnancy. Do not mix wine with fatty foods.

Folk Remedies:

1. **Arthritis (cold-type) with numbness and stiffness, neuralgia** – stir-fry dry black beans until the bean splits and they slightly burn; soak in good quality rice wine overnight. Filter and drink a small amount twice daily.
2. **Trauma and pain** – drink warm sake (rice wine), or other good quality wine for temporary relief.
3. **Menstrual pain** – drink wine that was prepared with the herb Motherwort (Leonorus cardiaca) prior to the onset of menses; the menstrual period will probably be a little heavier than usual.

Section Three

Remedies for Common Conditions

Conditions

Acne

This condition is characterized by skin blemishes or pimples. It can occur at any point throughout the lifetime and is often related to a hormonal imbalance. In Chinese terminology, the skin is controlled by the lungs, and acne is commonly a condition of heat in the lungs. Thus, the Chinese approach to this condition is to cool the heat, cleanse the lungs, and externally promote the healing process.

Recommendations: squash, cucumbers, watermelon, winter melon, celery, carrots, cabbage, beet tops, dandelions, aloe vera, mulberry leaf, carrot tops, lettuce, potato, cherries, papaya, pear, persimmon, raspberries, buckwheat, alfalfa sprouts, millet, brown rice, mung beans, plenty of water

Remedies:

1. Blend a cucumber, apply externally; leave on for twenty minutes then wash off.
2. Apply plain, low fat organic yogurt; leave on for twenty minutes then wash off.
3. Rub watermelon rind on the acne.
4. Apply aloe vera.
5. Eat watermelon or drink watermelon juice.
6. Drink dandelion and beet top tea.
7. Drink lukewarm water with two teaspoons of honey every morning on an empty stomach. This effectively lubricates the intestines. If one does not evacuate the intestines regularly, toxins either accumulate in the liver or erupt on the skin.
8. Boil raspberries to a concentrate and wash area with it.
9. Roast buckwheat, grind to a powder and mix with rice vinegar into a paste, then apply to area.
10. For oozing acne conditions, cover area with pearl barley powder overnight, wash off with water; or mix pearl

barley powder with aloe vera gel into a paste and leave on area overnight, then wash off with water.

11. Drink tea made from carrot tops, carrots, and beet tops.

12. For infected acne, apply a dandelion poultice to the area.

Avoid: fried foods, fatty or oily foods, spicy foods, coffee, alcohol, sugar, smoking, all stresses, constipation, makeup, washing with chemicals or soap (wash with cool water)*, chocolate, ice cream, soft drinks, dairy foods, red meat, shellfish, bamboo shoots, white mushrooms

If the face is dirty, steam it with hot water to induce sweating, then wash with cold water.

Acquired Immune Deficiency Syndrome (AIDS)

AIDS is a chronic retro-viral infection with the Human Immunodeficiency Virus (HIV) in a susceptible host, which produces severe defects in the cells. There is a reduction of part of the immune system called the Helper T cells. This leaves the patient vulnerable to many opportunistic infections and unusual cancers. The HIV virus is transmitted via sexual contact, exposure to infected blood, perinatal exposure or infected breast milk. Prominent symptoms include diarrhea, sweating, weight loss, neuropathy and wasting away. Aggressive infections like pneumonia and candidiasis can prove to be life threatening when AIDS compromises the immune system.

Recommendations: pearl barley, shiitake mushroom, ling zhi (ganoderma) mushroom, garlic, white and black fungus, brussel sprouts, bitter melon, squash, pumpkin, pumpkin seed, yam, apricot kernel, Chinese cucumber (Trichosanthes), water chestnut, mung bean, black bean, ginkgo nut, loquat, dandelion greens, egg yolk, jujube date, wild yam, green tea, daikon radish, lotus root, lotus seed, hawthorn berry

Remedies:

1. Make brown rice porridge with pearl barley, mung beans, yams and lotus seeds.

2. Soak dried shiitake mushrooms and/or white fungus, black fungus, and ling zhi mushrooms overnight. Boil for ten minutes in the soaking water. Then liquify in blender along with organic carrot tops. Drink on empty stomach daily.
3. Make tea from Chinese cucumber and jujube dates by simmering for thirty minutes. Drink three cups per day.
4. Make juice with fresh water chestnuts, lotus root, dandelion greens and fresh ginger.
5. Grind together apricot kernels, pumpkin seeds, nori seaweed, sesame seeds, cardamom and a pinch of salt. Use generously as seasoning over vegetables and grains.
6. Liquify fresh ginger root and aloe vera leaf (use only the soft center, peeling away the hard outer part). Drink one cup daily.
7. Consult a Chinese herbalist/acupuncturist for a Chinese herb formula.

Avoid: dairy, alcohol, coffee, sugar, fatty or fried foods, highly spiced foods, cold and raw foods, tomato, eggplant, bell peppers, shellfish

Allergies

An allergy is an acquired hypersensitivity to a substance that does not normally cause a body reaction. The allergenic substance may be pollen, smog, dust, certain chemicals in the air, chlorine, or certain food substances, which sometimes elicit a violent body response. This condition is characterized by nasal congestion, tearing, sneezing, wheezing, coughing, itching, skin rash and eruptions, dizziness and nausea.

Recommendations: ginger, onions, garlic, bamboo shoots, cabbage, beets, beet top tea, carrots, leafy greens, yams, organic chicken gizzards, ling zhi mushrooms

Remedies:

1. Drink ginger tea to induce sweating.

2. Drink beet top tea as a water source.

Avoid: wheat, citrus fruits, chocolate, shellfish, dairy products, eggs, potatoes, polluted meats, polluted air, and constipation

Anorexia and Bulimia

Anorexia is medically defined as a lack of appetite for food or a hysterical avoidance of food. This condition is particularly prevalent among young women obsessed with being thin. There is usually an extreme loss of weight, cessation of menstruation, fatigue, depression, and hypoglycemic patterns. Closely related to anorexia is bulimia, a condition in which one binges then purges, usually by vomiting. Emotional factors play a large part in both of these conditions.

Recommendations: bell pepper, cilantro, mustard greens, green onions, garlic, cinnamon, ginger, pumpkin, yam, beans, corn, barley, rice, persimmons, potatoes

Remedies:

1. For anorexia, prepare tea from green onions, garlic, cinnamon or ginger, to warm the stomach and stimulate digestive juices.
2. For anorexia, prepare soup from pumpkin, yam, beans, potatoes, corn, barley or vegetables.
3. For anorexia, prepare soupy rice.
4. For bulimia, give foods that bring rebellious Chi down, such as persimmons, cloves, potatoes, prune or plum tea, and mineral herbs such as oyster shell or mother of pearl shell tea.
5. For anorexia, dry fry bell pepper and black pepper.

Arthritis

Arthritis is an inflammation of the joints characterized by pain, redness, swelling, stiffness and hot sensation in the joints. Chinese medicine differentiates the following four types of arthritis: cold, wind, damp and hot. Often we observe two or three types of arthritis occurring simultaneously, such as cold and damp types together. In such cases, choose foods that aid each condition and are not contraindicated for either type. Herbal therapy can be of great benefit in clearing joints, improving circulation, and reducing pain. Acupuncture is one of the most effective treatments for arthritis, although progress is sometimes slow.

1. Cold Type Arthritis

This type is characterized by sharp, stabbing pain in a fixed location and coldness in the joints. The pain is relieved by heat such as a warming liniment, sunshine, or a heating pad. Usually, cold type individuals have a pale complexion.

Recommendations: garlic, green onions, pepper, black beans, sesame seeds, chicken, lamb, mustard greens, ginger, a small amount of rice wine if the individual does not have hypertension, spicy foods, grapes, parsnips, and 10-20 minutes of fresh air and sunshine daily

Remedies:

1. Rub garlic or ginger on the painful areas. Or moxa could be burned on a slice of ginger over the painful areas.
2. Drink scallion tea and rub on the painful areas.
3. Rub rice wine on the painful areas and drink one small glassful in the evening.
4. Drink grape vine tea added to red wine.
5. Make tea from parsnip, cinnamon, black pepper, and dried ginger.

Avoid: cold foods, raw foods, cold weather elements

2. Wind Type Arthritis

This type of arthritis is characterized by pain that shifts locations, comes and goes suddenly (much like the wind does), and sometimes causes dizziness.

Recommendations: nonpoisonous snake meat, scallions, grapes (not wine), grape vine and mulberry vine tea, black beans, most grains, and plenty of leafy vegetables

Avoid: meats, shellfish, sugar, alcohol, smoking, and all stimulants

3. Damp Type Arthritis

This type is characterized by heavy feeling extremities, stiffness, swelling, dull aching pain that lingers and sluggishness. Most obese people tend to be damp.

Recommendations: barley, mung beans, mustard greens, red beans, millet, sweet rice wine with meals, cornsilk tea, diuretic foods and herbs

Remedies:
1. Cook together barley, mung beans and red beans.
2. Drink cornsilk tea freely.

Avoid: cold foods, raw foods, and dairy products

4. Heat Type Arthritis

This is characterized by red, swollen, painful, hot joints, general disability and usually an acute onset.

Recommendations: plenty of fresh fruits and vegetables, dandelion, cabbage, mung beans, winter melon, soybean sprouts

Remedies:
1. Apply poultices of crushed dandelion greens, changing every two hours.

Avoid: spicy foods, green onions, alcohol, smoking, and all types of stress

Asthma

Asthma is characterized by wheezing or difficulty breathing due to the bronchials (branches) of the lungs becoming clogged with waste products, or constriction due to spasms, or swelling of the bronchials. Asthma may be triggered by an allergy to food, air pollution, cold air, heart weakness, previous lung damage, mental or physical fatigue, emotional disturbance, or hormonal imbalance. In the case of a weak heart, the heart is not strong enough to push the blood through the lungs to be oxygenated, and the blood flows back into the lungs. In this case there will also be edema and bruising as well.

Chinese medicine divides asthma into two types: the hot type characterized by rapid, coarse breathing, yellow, sticky mucus, fever, and red face; and the cold type characterized by white, clear, or foamy mucus, cold extremities, and pale face. The remedies listed would be useful for either type. During times of remission from asthma attacks, one would seek to nourish the lungs and kidneys.

Recommendations: apricot kernels, almonds, walnuts, basil, carrots, pumpkins, winter melon, sunflower seeds, loofa squash, figs, daikon, litchi (lychee) fruit, tangerines, loquats, honey, molasses, mustard greens, sesame seeds, placenta* and umbilical cord*

* *These substances are not easily obtainable in the United States. Only those from a healthy mother source are desirable.*

Remedies:

1. Egg yolk oil. This is made as follows: take 20 hard-boiled egg yolks; slowly heat in a dry pan, mashing them until the oil comes out. When the yolk has blackened, separate the egg yolk oil. Since it is very strong tasting, it is best taken in gelatin capsules, two after meals, three times daily. Continue this remedy for 15-30 days.
2. Mix ½ cup fig juice with ½ cup lukewarm water and drink daily.
3. Cut the top out of a small winter melon, remove the seeds, fill with molasses. Close the top with cheesecloth, and steam. Consume daily for seven days.

4. Take an unpeeled orange, pierce with a chopstick and roast until the peel blackens. Remove the peel and eat the fruit; one orange daily for seven days.
5. Bake squid bone until crisp; grind to a powder and take 1 teaspoon with honey daily for seven days.
6. Drink apricot kernel tea.
7. Drink fresh fig juice three times daily.

Avoid: mucus producing foods, cold foods, fruits, salads, all shellfish, dairy products, watermelon, bananas, mung beans, salty foods, cold weather, and especially ice cream

Cancer

According to Chinese Medicine, cancer is an abnormal growth of tissue that results from stagnation of Chi, blood, mucus, or body fluids. The stagnation can be caused by an external irritant such as cigarette smoke or chemical-laden foods, or by strong emotions. When the body is irritated over a long period of time, it reacts to the irritant by producing cells to protect itself. However, at certain point the cell growth becomes abnormal and uncontrollable and cancer cells result. Strong emotions lead to Chi stagnation which in turn can lead to stagnation of blood, mucus or body fluids.

The Western approach to cancer is to kill the cancer cells with harsh chemicals, radiation, or surgery. However, these methods also harm healthy cells. The Chinese approach to cancer is to support the body so that it can combat the cancer cells by itself. Because cancer is considered to be a toxin in the body, a detoxifying diet is also utilized.

Recommendations: seaweed, shiitake mushrooms, figs, beet tops, papayas, mung beans, licorice, sea cucumbers, carrots, garlic, walnuts, litchi (lychee) fruits, mulberries, asparagus, pumpkins, burdock, dandelion greens, white fungus, taro roots, pearl barley, grains, plenty of fresh fruits and vegetables

Remedies:
1. Blend shiitake or ling zhi mushrooms and white fungus, boil and drink the soup three times daily.
2. Boil together mung beans, pearl barley, azuki beans, and figs. This makes a delicious dessert that will aid appetite and sustain energy level.
3. Make tea from dandelion, burdock, and chrysanthemum flowers; you may also add beet tops or carrot tops. Drink this as the regular beverage every day.
4. Always wash commercially grown fruits and vegetables in salt water to neutralize chemicals.
5. Eat garlic and seaweed, slightly stir-fried in water.
6. Drink carrot and celery juice.
7. Make blender juice from a mixture of fresh vegetables and drink warm.
8. For breast cancer, make tea from asparagus and dandelion and apply poultice to breast.
9. For breast tumor, charcoal the pumpkin cap into powder; take one teaspoon of powder in one small glass of rice wine twice daily.
10. Make tea from seaweed (any variety), peach kernel and green orange peels.
11. For externally visible tumors, make a poultice from seaweed, ginger and dandelion, and apply locally.

Avoid: meat (if patient cannot tolerate a vegetarian diet, a little fish can be eaten), chicken, coffee, cinnamon, anise, pepper, dairy products, spicy foods (except garlic), high-fat foods, cooked oils, chemical additives, moldy foods, smoking, constipation, stress, and all irritations

Candida Yeast Infection

This condition is becoming fairly common in modern society, primarily due to the widespread, long-term use of antibiotics which severely weakens the immune system. Everyone has candida yeast living in our bodies; only when disharmony and weakness occur do systemic yeast infections develop. The symptoms include chronic fatigue, chronic infections (primarily in the skin, bowels, bladder, vagina, and throat), diarrhea or constipation, headaches, bloating, and poor digestion. When the immune system is weakened because of overwork, excessive sex, or stress, the candida flares up and the body can no longer control it. In the case of AIDS, candida infection can become life threatening.

Recommendation: dandelions, beet tops, carrot tops, barley, garlic, rice vinegar, mung beans, citrus fruits

Avoid: sugar, excessive fruits, and yeast containing foods, processed foods, cheese, fermented foods, soy sauce, smoking, alcohol, caffeine and constipation

Cataracts

This condition usually affects older people. The lens of the eye becomes cloudy and visual acuity is decreased. It may be accompanied by dizziness, vertigo, fatigue, and lower back pain. Western medicine treats cataracts by surgically removing the lens.

Recommendations: chrysanthemum, cilantro, spinach, cloves, water chestnuts, yams, goji berries, black beans. Exercise the eyes regularly and get plenty of oxygen into the bloodstream.

Remedies:

1. Stuff nose with fresh cilantro and inhale the aroma. Do this three times daily.
2. Cook spinach with no spices and eat daily.
3. Steam the eyes over boiling spinach.
4. Grind cloves into a very fine powder and add a little milk to make an ointment. Apply to eyes 3-5 times daily.
5. Make fresh water chestnut juice and use as an eye drop.

6. Make tea from clam shells, orange peels, goji berries, and chrysanthemum. Drink three times daily for at least two weeks.
7. Mash together black beans, sesame seeds, yams, and walnuts. Then add a little honey and eat one tablespoon of the mixture twice daily for one month.

Avoid: any type of spices (very important), salt, garlic, eye-strain, constipation

Chronic Bladder Infection

This is a common condition in women, characterized by painful or burning urination, the feeling that urine remains in the bladder after urinating, fever and low backache. If this condition occurs in a man it is a warning sign of something more serious such as venereal disease or cancer. Women are prone to chronic bladder infections because of the short length of their urethras. In Chinese terminology it is a condition of damp heat.

Recommendations: watermelon, cranberry, blueberry, pears, carrots, celery, corn, mung beans, cornsilk, squash, wheat, water chestnuts, barley, red beans, millet, cantaloupe, grapes, strawberries, lotus roots, loquats, plenty of water, cooling and diuretic foods in general.

Remedies:
1. Drink watermelon and pear juice three times daily.
2. Drink carrot and celery juice three times daily.
3. Drink cornsilk tea freely.
4. Eat squash soup for at least seven days.
5. Eat steamed lotus root and water chestnuts twice daily.
6. Drink blended mung bean juice.
7. Drink fresh strawberry or unsweetend cranberry juice.
8. Drink tea made from wheat and pearl barley.

Avoid: heavy proteins, meat, dairy products, onions, scallions, ginger, black pepper, alcohol

Chronic Bronchitis

This is a common condition in older people, often due to a low-ered immune system. It often occurs during winter and spring. Main symptoms include cough, mucus, shortness of breath, and a feeling of fullness in the chest.

Recommendations: carrots, apricot kernels, persimmons, white fungus, pears, honey, jellyfish, ginger, water chest-nuts, yams, sweet potatoes, Chinese red or black dates, daikon radish, walnuts, papaya, peach kernels, lotus root, seaweed, betel nut, white pepper, loquat leaves, lily bulbs, pine nuts, mulberry leaves, chrysanthemum, ginko nuts, basil seeds, pumpkins, taro, winter melon seeds. Always try to keep warm.

Remedies:
1. Cook carrots and apricot kernels in rice porridge. Eat three times daily for one month.
2. Take white fungus and rock sugar, steam and eat 2-3 times daily for one month.
3. Remove cores of 2-3 pears and fill with honey, eat before bed every day for one month.
4. Blend together jellyfish and water chestnut to make soup.
5. Mash together ginger, apricot kernels, pine nuts, and walnuts; add rock sugar, and steam. Eat 2-3 tablespoons twice daily for at least two weeks.
6. Make juice from pineapple and lemon; drink before meals for immediate relief.
7. Boil three dried persimmons in two cups of water, re-duced to one cup. Add some honey and drink 2-3 times daily.
8. Add maltose to daikon radish and steam. Eat 2-3 times daily for relief within one week.
9. Peel a papaya, add some honey, steam and eat.
10. Grind seaweed into powder, add honey and make into small pills. Take one teaspoon of pills 2-3 times daily after meals.

11. Boil tea from betel nuts, drink as your water for one month.
12. Make a tea from carrots, white pepper, ginger, and dried orange peels. Drink two cups daily.
13. Warm one tablespoon each of honey and sesame oil, in a pan and take for immediate relief.
14. Cut banana into small pieces and cook with rock sugar until sugar melts. Eat 1-2 pieces of banana every evening for one week.
15. Use seed from such vegetables as daikon, basil, spinach, and make tea, adding honey.
16. Take one tablespoon molasses and ½ tablespoon raw ginger juice with warm water 2-3 times daily.
17. Use fresh, yellow chrysanthemum flowers and boil into a thick juice; take regularly.
18. Mash cooked taro root and add honey.
19. Drink raw eggplant juice (especially good for blood in the mucus).

Avoid: overworking, getting chilled, stimulating foods, spicy foods, smoking, alcohol, caffeine, cold drinks

Chronic Fatigue Syndrome

This syndrome consists of a set of variable symptoms including chronic or recurrent fatigue, sore throat, tender lymph nodes, headaches, muscle pains, and general depression. Often the patient has flu-like symptoms that extend for a long period of time. Most chronic fatigue patients are observed to have undergone prolonged stress, repeated infections, and often become overwhelmed by life's simple demands. Conditions like herpes, candida and hypoglycemia compound the situation. The patient is advised to seek lifestyle corrections such as reducing stress, resting more, and gentle exercise.

Recommendations: winter melon, pumpkins, pumpkin seeds, yams, sweet potatoes, lima beans, black beans, soybeans, strawberries, watermelon, azuki beans, pineapple, chestnuts, papaya, figs, garlic, onions, scallions, ginger, daikon radish, pearl barley, lotus seed, white fungus, egg white, cabbage, carrots, pears, organic chicken, mung beans, buckwheat, jujube dates

Remedies:
1. Eat frequent, small meals and drink more liquids.
2. Juice and drink daily: fresh water chestnut, lotus root, pear, watermelon, and carrots.
3. Make soup from lotus seed, white fungus and figs.
4. Chop garlic finely and stir-fry with egg white, parsley and diced yams.
5. Make soup from cabbage, azuki beans, winter melon and pumpkin.
6. Make chicken soup with garlic, onions, scallions, ginger and daikon radish. Drink soup or cook rice porridge with the broth.
7. Make buckwheat and rice porridge with chestnuts and longan fruit (Euphoria longan).

Avoid: dairy products, alcohol, coffee, sugar, fatty or fried foods, overly spicy foods, cold and raw foods, tomato, eggplant, bell pepper, shellfish

Chronic Sinus Infection

This condition is due to an acute inflammation of the nasal passages over a long period of time. There is often drainage or congestion, difficulty breathing through the nose, sometimes dryness of the nostrils, headaches, and ringing in the ears.

Recommendations: ginger, green onions, magnolia flower, bananas, garlic, black mushrooms, chrysanthemum flowers, mulberry leaves, apricot kernels. Get plenty of fresh air.

Remedies:
1. Make tea from magnolia flower, basil, ginger, and green onion. Drink three times daily for at least one week.
2. Combine magnolia flowers and eggs, cook and eat.

3. Make tea from mulberry leaves and chrysanthemums, then cook rice porridge in the tea, adding apricot kernels.
4. Mash green onions, soak cotton balls and alternately put in nostrils after having washed them with salt water.
5. Mix garlic juice and olive oil, soak cotton balls with mixture and alternately put in nostrils after having washed them with salt water.
6. Cook black mushrooms into a concentrated soup, then slowly use a dropper to put drops in the nose.
7. Boil tea of mint, basil, and ginger. While boiling the tea, inhale the steam through the nose, three times daily for at least two months.

Avoid: extremes of exposure to weather elements, coffee, smoking, stress, picking the nose, polluted air and smog

Common Cold

There are two basic types or stages of colds. In Chinese terminology they are the wind cold type and the wind heat type. They have different symptoms and different treatments.

1. Wind cold type

This type often occurs during a change in the weather or when one is exposed to wind and cold. With a weak immune function, these pathogens enter the skin. The symptoms could include chills, fever, no sweating, headache, body ache, stiff neck, and clear copious nasal discharge. This is often the first stage of a cold. When the pathogens are at this initial, superficial stage, we seek to sweat them out. A hot bath or dry sauna could be beneficial to begin the sweating process.

Recommendations: ginger, garlic, mustard greens and seeds, grapefruit peel, cilantro, parsnip, scallions, cinnamon, basil, soupy rice porridge, and eating as little as possible so as not to burden the body with a lot of digestion

Remedies:
1. Lightly boil for five minutes the following: garlic, ginger, green onion, basil, mustard, or cinnamon. Drink the tea; go to bed and prepare to sweat.
2. Drink cilantro and ginger tea.
3. Drink scallion and basil tea.
4. Make tea from dried grapefruit peel.
5. Make tea from mustard greens, cilantro and green onion.
6. Make tea from parsnip and ginger.

Avoid: shellfish, heavy proteins and fats, meats and all vinegars. Vinegar closes the pores and "traps the thief in the house."

2. Wind heat type

This type of common cold is characterized by high fever, some chills, sweating, sore throat, cough, headache, body ache, and yellow nasal discharge or sputum.

Recommendations: mint, cabbage, chrysanthemum flowers, burdock root, cilantro, dandelion, apples, pears, bitter melon, drink plenty of fluids and get plenty of rest

Remedies:
1. Drink cabbage broth freely.
2. Drink cilantro and mint tea.
3. Drink mint, chrysanthemum and dandelion tea.
4. Drink mint, dandelion and licorice tea.
5. Drink burdock tea.

Avoid: shellfish, meats, vinegar, drafts, and hot foods

Constipation

Constipation is a lack of regular evacuation of the bowels or difficulty in defecation. The resulting symptoms may include bloating, abdominal pain, abdominal hardness, and bad breath. We should evacuate at least once daily, with the optimal times energetically being from 5:00 a.m.-7:00 a.m. The longer the waste remains in the intestines, the drier it gets and the more difficult to pass. Food takes about 6-8 hours to go from the mouth to the intestines. Strained evacuation leads to hemorrhoids. Regular enemas or colonics are not a healthy solution to the problem. It is best to set a certain time for evacuation and train the body to respond accordingly. Rubbing the belly in a clockwise direction 100 times can stimulate peristalsis. Breathing with the mouth open is also beneficial in stimulating a bowel movement

Recommendations: bananas, apples, walnuts, figs, spinach, peaches, pears, pine nuts, sesame seeds, mulberries, grapefruit, yams, honey, azuki beans, apricot kernel, milk, yogurt, alfalfa sprouts, beets, cabbage, bok choy, cauliflower, potato, Chinese cabbage, salt water

Remedies:
1. Eat two bananas on an empty stomach, followed by a glass of water.
2. Drink a glass of lukewarm water with 2 teaspoons of honey on an empty stomach.
3. Drink blended beets and cabbage on an empty stomach.
4. Make beet soup.
5. Eat 5-10 figs on an empty stomach, followed by a glass of water.
6. Drink a glass of lukewarm water with 2 teaspoons of salt, on an empty stomach. This remedy should be used as a last resort when nothing else has worked and should not be used by those with edema or hypertension.
7. Eat a fresh apple on an empty stomach.
8. Drink mulberry juice.
9. Eat lightly steamed asparagus and cabbage at night before retiring.

Avoid: stress, tension, spicy foods, fried foods and meat

Coronary Heart Disease

This is a condition in which the arteries that supply the heart become hardened and clogged, eventually leading to deprivation of oxygen and nourishment to the heart, thereby causing heart attack. Recent research has attributed the cause of coronary heart disease to faulty diet, obesity, continuous stress and tension, mental fatigue, hypertension, diabetes, low thyroid function, and smoking. Typical symptoms with coronary heart disease are dizziness, vertigo, palpitations, chest fullness, shortness of breath, pain in the chest area, irregular heart beat, spontaneous sweating, hardness in the lips and tongue, and angina pain when there is an obstruction.

Recommendations: American ginseng, brown rice, black fungus, sea cucumber, Chinese black dates, peanuts, vinegar, shiitake mushrooms, celery, seaweed, cassia seeds, lotus roots, jellyfish, chrysanthemums, hawthorn berries, water chestnuts, mung beans, pearl barley, peach kernels, ginger, soy sprouts, mung sprouts, other sprouts, wheat bran, buckwheat, persimmons, bananas, watermelon, sunflower seeds, lotus seeds, black sesame seeds, wheat, garlic, green tea

Remedies:
1. Take three grams American ginseng and cook with one cup brown rice and some rock sugar. Cook into a porridge and consume every morning.
2. Soak black fungus and black mushrooms overnight, then steam one hour; eat before bedtime.
3. Steam together the following: sea cucumber, Chinese black dates. Eat every morning on an empty stomach.
4. Soak 10-15 peanuts in rice vinegar for 24 hours and consume both the peanuts and the rice vinegar in the morning.
5. Cook tea from white or button mushrooms and Chinese black dates. Drink twice daily for one month.
6. Make tea from seaweed, cassia seeds, and lotus root. Drink the tea and eat the seaweed and lotus root twice daily for at least one month.

7. Combine jellyfish, water chestnut, and rice vinegar; cook together into a soup.
8. Cook celery and yellow squash soup and eat once a day for at least twenty days.
9. Make tea from chrysanthemum flowers, hawthorn berries, and cassia seeds. Drink one cup three times daily for at least twenty days.
10. Take black fungus, pearl barley, and dried orange peel and boil into a soup.
11. Grind betel nut and hawthorn berries; add rice flour, stir together and steam. Eat often.
12. Take one tablespoon honey three times daily.
13. Steam soy and alfalfa sprouts together and add some rice vinegar.
14. Slightly roast wheat and oat bran with black sesame and sunflower seeds. Sprinkle on vegetables or porridge.
15. Drink at least two cups green tea every day.
16. Go on a watermelon fast for three consecutive days.
17. Take peach kernels, safflowers, hawthorn berries, and make tea. Drink two cups daily for at least one month.

Avoid: fatty foods, stimulating foods, spicy foods, coffee, smoking, alcohol, simple carbohydrates (sugar, white flour), salt, stress, tension, worrying, emotional stimulation, lack of sleep

Diabetes

Diabetes is characterized by a high level of sugar in the blood and urine. Symptoms include excessive thirst, hunger, and urination. The Chinese refer to this condition as *exhaustion syndrome*. Proper exercise is of utmost importance in stimulating normal glandular functions; exercises such as tai chi chuan, chi gong or the Taoist Eight Treasures are particularly valuable (visit www.taoofwellness.com for DVDs and books).

Recommendations: pumpkin, wheat, mung beans, winter melon, celery, pears, spinach, yams, peas, sweet rice, soybeans, tofu, mulberries, squash, daikon radish, cabbage, organic pig or chicken pancreas

Remedies:
1. Eat a slice of pumpkin with each meal.
2. Make pumpkin and yam pie with no sweeteners.
3. Prepare soup from cabbage, yam, winter melon, and lentils.
4. Drink daikon, celery, carrot, and spinach juice.
5. Steam tofu, cool to room temperature, add sesame oil and slices of raw squash.
6. Make soup from mung beans, peas, and barley.
7. Drink chrysanthemum tea whenever thirsty.
8. Eat non-sweetened sweet rice cake or mochi between meals.
9. Steam millet with yam and a few dates.

Avoid: sweets, sugar, honey, molasses, smoking, alcohol, caffeine, spicy foods and most raw fruits

Diarrhea

This is characterized by the frequent passage of abnormally watery stools, usually caused by increased peristalsis, irritation of the intestines through improper diet, drugs, bacterial infections, parasites, or worms. This differs from dysentery in that diarrhea is generally due to digestive weakness, biological imbalance, and in general is a chronic condition. Dysentery, on the other hand, is caused by an infectious condition.

Recommendations: garlic, black pepper, blueberries, cinnamon, raspberry leaves, lotus seeds, burned rice, yams, sweet potatoes, fresh fig leaves, peas, buckwheat, litchi, guava peel, apples, charcoaled bread, ginger, pearl barley, basil, unripe prunes

Remedies:
1. Cook rice porridge with lotus seed and yam or with barley.

2. Eat burnt rice or bread.
3. Make tea from dried litchi and Chinese black date.
4. Take two tablespoons dried apples, three times daily on an empty stomach with warm water.
5. Cook rice porridge with ginger and black pepper.
6. Drink black tea.
7. Take two bulbs of garlic, bake until black. Then boil in water and drink the tea.
8. Make tea from guava peel.
9. Make tea from ginger, fennel, basil, and Chinese black dates.
10. Make tea from unripe prunes.
11. Eat sweet rice porridge.

Avoid: cold, raw foods, most fruits, juices, overeating

Dysentery

Dysentery is a condition of intestinal inflammation characterized by abdominal pain, intense, urgent, watery diarrhea with foul smelling, bloody or mucous feces, dry mouth, thirst, and decreased urination. To prevent dehydration, plenty of fluids should be consumed. The person will sometimes defecate 30 or 40 times daily. Food poisoning can be a possible cause. Dysentery is considered to be contagious and is usually transmitted through unsanitary food or water. Sometimes the person also has vomiting.

Recommendations: buckwheat, sweet potatoes, peas, celery, scallions, taro root, ginger, garlic, carrots, daikon radish, green pepper, winter melon, cantaloupe, bitter melon, hawthorn berries, figs, Chinese prunes, pears, persimmons, guavas, olives, sunflower seeds, lotus roots, tea, soy products, corn, pumpkins, water chestnuts, squash, honey, mung beans, cherries, pineapples, watermelon, brown rice, oats, chicken eggs (only if chronic)

Remedies:
1. Take carrot juice mixed with a little ginger juice, honey, and green tea; drink one cup daily.
2. Make mung bean soup and drink throughout the day.
3. Stir-fry ginger, garlic, celery and peas together; incorporate into regular diet.
4. Eat four persimmons daily.
5. Soak Chinese prunes in rice wine for three days; take 10 prunes twice daily.
6. Make sweet potato and pumpkin mush and have three times a day; for breakfast, lunch, and dinner.
7. Steam black fungus with a little sugar in about 1- ½ cups of water.
8. Charcoal dried ginger, powder it, and take one teaspoon with soupy rice.
9. Drink sour prune tea before meals on an empty stomach.
10. Drink plum peel tea.
11. Cook brown rice with persimmon cap and consume the rice.
12. Consume eggs cooked with rice vinegar. This remedy is only appropriate for chronic cases of dysentery.

Avoid: dairy products, eggs, high-fiber foods, hard to digest foods, fried foods, meats, fish, raw foods, cold foods, chicken eggs (in acute cases of dysentery)

Eczema

This is a common skin condition that often affects extremities, genitalia, as well as other parts. The skin lesion is characterized by a raised spot that turns into a blister and eventually erupts, ulcerates and then forms a scab which is later sloughed off. It can cause extreme itching and pain.

Recommendations: potatoes, broccoli, dandelion, mung beans, seaweed, pearl barley, azuki beans, cornsilk, water chestnuts, winter melon, watermelon

Remedies:
1. Mash fresh potato and apply locally, changing every four hours, for three days.
2. Apply honey to area.
3. Apply mashed daikon radish to area.
4. Make tea from mung beans and pearl barley and drink.
5. Make tea from dandelion and cornsilk.
6. Make tea from azuki beans, pearl barley, and cornsilk. Drink tea and eat the solids three times daily.
7. Boil soup from seaweed and winter melon, drinking at least once a day for ten days.
8. Externally, wash with equal portions of salt and borax, dissolved in warm water; wash area 2-3 times daily.
9. Make tea from lily bulbs, Chinese black dates, and mulberries, drink three times daily for at least ten days.

Avoid: external stimulation such as extreme weather conditions of wind, cold, dampness, dryness, heat, excessive sun exposure, chemical exposure. Use clean water to bathe; avoid soap.

Edema/Swelling

Edema is a condition of swelling due to abnormal accumulation of fluids in the cells. It can occur anywhere in the body, however, the common places that edema occurs are face, lower extremities, and abdomen. Abdominal edema can cause ascites and is usually related to liver dysfunction, such as cirrhosis of the liver. The treatment is chosen to promote diuresis and ease urination. Heart, kidney, and lungs are the organs that may be involved.

Recommendations: red azuki beans, corn, ginger skin, winter melon, winter melon skin, squash, apples, mulberries, peaches, tangerines, coconuts, seaweed, fish, celery, green onions, garlic, bamboo shoots, spinach, water chestnuts, millet, wheat, black beans, pearl barley, carrots, watermelon, oats, beef

Remedies:
1. Take fish, preferably carp, and cook into soup with azuki beans. Use ten cups of water and cook down to one cup; consume only the liquid.
2. Take winter melon rind and azuki beans and enough water to cover; cook and eat three times daily.
3. Drink blended juice of apple, carrot, and green onion twice daily.
4. Boil tea made from ginger skin.
5. Cook together pearl barley, mung beans, and azuki beans into a soup; consume three times daily. You may also add black beans to this soup.
6. Daily diet should be bland and should include plenty of vegetables and fish.
7. Eat plenty of watermelon in the summer.
8. Drink coconut juice daily.
9. Cook oats and mung beans to a mash and consume until swelling subsides.
10. Consume soupy pearl barley.
11. Drink beef stew broth.
12. Drink tea made from watermelon rind.

Avoid: rich foods, salty foods, lamb, stimulating foods, wine, garlic, pepper, shellfish, fatty foods, and greasy foods

Glaucoma

This is a disease characterized by an increase in the pressure inside of the eye. Its onset can be either acute or chronic. The sufferer often complains that lights have halos around them. The condition can progress to a point in which the pressure causes atrophy of the optic nerve, leading to blindness. During the onset, there may be pain, headaches, nausea, vomiting, and blurry vision.

Recommendations: chrysanthemum, mint, oyster shells, mulberries, black sesame seeds, betel nuts, goji berries, cassia seeds, grapefruit, lemons, oranges, carrots, beets, beet tops

Remedies:
1. Boil tea from mulberries, oyster shell, and black sesame seeds; drink three times daily.
2. Make tea from chrysanthemum and mint; drink twice daily.
3. Boil tea from betel nut; drink twice daily.
4. Boil tea from cassia seeds, orange peels, beets, and goji berries; then use the tea to cook rice porridge; add a little honey.

Avoid: Self-treatment is not recommended due to the seriousness of this condition. Seek professional guidance for close observation of the condition. Avoid visual stimulation, stimulating foods, alcohol, drugs, smoking, coffee, salt, drinking too much water

Headache

There are many different types of headaches, such as migraines and headaches caused by muscular tension, hypertension, common cold, mental stress, hormonal changes, and eye strain. Each type of headache has a corresponding treatment.

Recommendations: chrysanthemum flowers, mint, green onions, ginger, oyster shells, pearl barley, carrots, prunes, buckwheat, peach kernels

Remedies for headaches due to common cold or flu:
1. Make tea from ginger and green onions, boiling for five minutes; drink and try to sweat.
2. Steam aching portion of head over mint and cinnamon tea that is cooking, then dry head afterwards, avoiding drafts.
3. Make tea from chrysanthemum flowers, cassia seeds and drink.
4. Make buckwheat meal into a paste and apply to painful area until it sweats.
5. Drink green tea.

6. Make rice porridge and add garlic and green onions. Eat while hot, then get under covers and sweat.

Remedies for headaches due to high blood pressure, menstrual cycles, emotional stress or tension, or migraines:

1. Make carrot juice. If headache is on left side, squirt carrot juice into left nostril; if only right side, squirt into right nostril; if both sides are painful, squirt into both nostrils.
2. Take lemon juice and ½ tablespoon baking soda mixed in a glass of water and drink.
3. Make tea of Chinese prunes, mint, and green tea.
4. Make tea of oyster shells and chrysanthemum flowers, slowly boiling the shells for 1 ½ hours, then adding the flowers for the last 30 minutes.
5. Mash peach kernels and walnuts, mix with rice wine and lightly roast it; take two tablespoons three times daily.
6. Rinse head with warm water, gradually increasing the temperature to hot.

Avoid: spicy food, lack of sleep, alcohol, smoking, excessive stimulation, eye strain, stress

For menstrual-type headaches, please see section on Premenstrual Syndrome (PMS).

Hemorrhoids

This common condition is related to constipation. With dry stools, the person strains to move the bowels which causes friction on delicate rectal tissues. Sometimes it can cause bleeding. Hemorrhoids can be due to over-consumption of alcohol, spicy or fried foods, lack of exercise, sitting or standing too long, too much sex, pregnancy, or chronic constipation. A hemorrhoid is a varicose vein in the rectum and can be very painful.

Recommendations: sea cucumber, black fungus, water chestnut, buckwheat, tangerines, figs, plums, fish, prunes, guavas, bamboo shoots, mung beans, winter melon, black sesame seeds, persimmons, bananas, squash, cucumbers, taro, tofu, cooling foods

Remedies:
1. Soak lower body in a warm bath to which has been added the tea of either mugwort (Artemsia argyi), carrot tops or figs. Bath should be warm enough to induce sweating and done daily.
2. Take black fungus with rice every morning for breakfast on an empty stomach; do this for one month.
3. Steam sea cucumber without salt or spices and eat for immediate pain relief.
4. Roast and grind black sesame seeds; take with warm water and honey every night before retiring.
5. Steam dried persimmons and eat.
6. Wash hemorrhoid with winter melon tea.
7. Boil papaya tea for two hours, without the skin, soak the area.
8. Grind mung bean powder, boil with dandelion greens and wash area with the tea.
9. Steam figs; add honey and steam again several times, until it becomes soggy; consume every day.
10. Insert a raw potato suppository after each bowel movement.
11. Eat a banana every day on an empty stomach.

The following remedies are used for bleeding hemorrhoids:
1. Cook black fungus with brown sugar; consume daily.
2. Eat three bananas with some honey on an empty stomach every morning.
3. Eat a fresh squash before breakfast and after dinner everyday for two weeks.

4. Make taro root soup and eat regularly until bleeding stops and hemorrhoid heals.
5. Mash fresh plums and take with lukewarm water three times daily.
6. Wash area with hot water, then apply a cotton ball that has been soaked in garlic juice. Change cotton ball every hour.

Avoid: stimulating foods, spicy foods, alcohol, smoking, constipation, stress, lack of exercise, standing or sitting too long

Hepatitis

Hepatitis is a liver condition that can be caused by many drugs and toxic agents, as well as by numerous viruses. The manifestations include jaundice, anorexia, nausea, vomiting, malaise, fever, tender liver area, and flu-like symptoms. Upon examination of the blood, the liver enzymes are abnormally high. Viral Hepatitis A is generally transmitted via the fecal-oral route, whereas viral Hepatitis B and C is transmitted via blood and sexual fluids. Bed rest is necessary in the initial stages. Hepatitis B and C can become chronic.

Recommendations: rice, barley, millet, azuki bean, pearl barley, squash, cucumber, grapefruit, ling zhi mushroom, cornsilk, dandelion greens, beet greens, pears, water chestnut, carrot, cabbage, spinach, celery, winter melon, rice vinegar, apple, orange, pineapple, lotus root, watermelon

Remedies:
1. Cook lotus root and puree, then cook into rice or millet porridge.
2. Make tea from cornsilk, dandelion and beet greens. Drink regularly as a beverage.
3. Juice watermelon, celery and pears.
4. Make mung bean soup with pearl barley.
5. Soak grapefruit and peel in rice vinegar overnight, then take one teaspoon in one cup of warm liquid.

6. Make tea from ling zhi mushrooms and jujube dates.
7. Take cucumber juice on empty stomach every morning.
8. Charcoal grapefruit peel and take ½ teaspoon with rice water after every meal.
9. Make soup from winter melon and kabocha squash.

Avoid: dairy products, alcohol, coffee, sugar, fatty and fried foods, overly spicy foods, cold and raw foods, tomato, eggplant, bell peppers, shellfish

Hives

Hives is a skin condition which is characterized by an intermittent attack of extreme itching which results in welts, primarily on the arms, legs, back and face. These elevated spots can spread throughout the entire body with scratching. Hives may be brought on by an exposure to an allergen or after consumption of shellfish. This condition in Chinese Medicine is considered an invasion of wind.

Recommendations: winter melon rind, chrysanthemum, vinegar, papaya, ginger, Chinese black dates, dried prunes, black sesame seeds, black beans, litchi, pearl barley, cornsilk, soybeans, mung beans, licorice, hawthorn berries, peach kernels, maple leaves, shiitake mushrooms, mint

Remedies:
1. Externally, take a sea salt bath, rubbing salt on the hives.
2. Boil a thick tea from fresh maple leaves for an external wash of hives.
3. Internally, drink tea made from 15 grams gypsum, 9 grams hawthorn berries, 60 grams black beans, some winter melon rind and chrysanthemum flowers. Add some honey and drink three times daily.
4. Cook together papaya, ginger and rice vinegar until vinegar dries up. Eat the ginger and papaya twice daily for at least ten days.
5. Mix honey with rice wine and steam. Drink two tablespoons on an empty stomach every morning.

6. Cook together black sesame seeds, black beans, and Chinese black dates and eat at least once daily.
7. Make tea of dried litchi, add some brown sugar and drink three times daily.
8. Make tea of lotus seeds and ½ teaspoon pearl powder.
9. Make tea of cornsilk and pearl barley and drink twice daily for at least ten days.
10. Take equal portions of mung and soybeans, grind into powder, add water and boil fifteen minutes. Then strain and drink one cup twice daily.
11. Make tea of licorice, mung beans, and gypsum, drink three times daily for at least three days.
12. Eat 2-3 dried prunes daily.

Avoid: shellfish, allergic foods

Hypertension

Hypertension, or high blood pressure, is characterized by a wiry and rapid pulse, headache, dizziness, tinnitus, blurry vision, palpitations, chest tightness or fullness, fatigue, insomnia, vertigo and numbness of the extremities. It is commonly caused by hardening of the arteries, kidney dysfunction, or liver dysfunction. The normal range of blood pressure is between 100-135 mmHg for the systolic measurement and 70-85 mmHg for the diastolic measurement.

Recommendations: celery, spinach, garlic, bananas, sunflower seeds, honey, tofu, mung beans, bamboo shoots, seaweed, vinegar, tomatoes, water chestnuts, corn, apples, persimmons, peas, buckwheat, jellyfish, watermelon, hawthorn berries, eggplant, plums, mushrooms, lemons, lotus root, chrysanthemum, cassia seeds

Remedies:
1. Drink warm celery juice three times daily.
2. Eat two raw tomatoes on an empty stomach every day for a month.

3. Drink water, vinegar and honey regularly.
4. Drink chrysanthemum and spinach tea regularly.
5. Drink cornsilk tea.
6. Sleep on a pillow of chrysanthemum flowers to draw heat out of the head.
7. Make mung bean soup.
8. Take garlic oil capsules to clean out the arteries. The capsules have the advantage of not overly stimulating the taste buds in the warming direction. The taste buds start the functions of many physiological processes; the spicy flavor can be too stimulating, in general for hyper-sensitive individuals.
9. Steam or bake jellyfish about twelve minutes; add vinegar, soy sauce, and sesame oil. Take daily for about two months.
10. Steam tofu, cool to room temperature, add vinegar and sesame oil This can be combined with soupy rice for a nutritious breakfast.
11. Make lotus root tea and drink three cups daily for one month.
12. Make tea from chrysanthemum flowers and cassia seeds and drink daily.
13. Steam white fungus for two hours and take before bedtime.
14. Drink hawthorn berry tea continuously for a long period of time.
15. Make soup from abalone and seaweed.
16. During the summer months, make watermelon juice or eat watermelon every day.
17. Make tea from watermelon rind, mugwort, and mulberry branches, drink three cups daily for two months.
18. Take celery, white onion (sweet), garlic, water chestnuts, tomatoes and four cups water; boil down to one cup and drink every night before bed.

19. Make soup using seaweed, pearl barley and a little honey; eat every day for five days.
20. Mix pig bile and mung bean powder; take one teaspoon daily for at least eight days.
21. Eat soup of black or white mushrooms daily.
22. Eat three apples daily.
23. Drink organic banana peel tea.
24. Make tea from one peeled lemon, ten fresh water chestnuts, and 2 ½ cups water.
25. Drink three glasses daily of unripened persimmon juice for one week.

Avoid: smoking, alcohol, spicy foods, coffee, caffeine, all stimulants, fatty or fried foods, salty foods, stress, constipation, potatoes, strong emotions, pork, overeating, and low levels of calcium* in the body

* *For low calcium levels, make tea made from shells (oyster, abalone, mother of pearl) or fossils (dragon bones and teeth); strain and drink.*

Hypoglycemia

This very common condition is due to a stressful lifestyle and a heavily sugar laden diet. Hypoglycemia is characterized by low blood sugar, chronic fatigue, nervousness, shakiness, headaches, fatigue when hungry, irritability or faintness if a meal is late, sweet cravings, waking at night hungry, night sweats, light-headedness, mood swings, depression and difficulty concentrating.

Recommendations: sweet rice, brown rice, yams, potatoes, walnuts, tofu, soybeans, corn, fish, chicken, vegetables, black beans, nuts (a good snack between meals), mild exercise, regular meal schedule, 4-5 small meals daily

Avoid: simple carbohydrates such as white flour and sugar, honey, fructose, maple syrup, sweet fruits (eat very sparingly), coffee, smoking, fatty or fried foods, and all stimulants

Impotence

This is a weak condition, most likely due to a nervous weakness, excessive stress, worrying, tension, physical fatigue, frequent masturbation, or excessive indulgence in sex. Impotence is characterized by not being able to have an erection when there is a desire to have intercourse, and there may be premature ejaculation. Other symptoms may include dizziness, insomnia, excessive dreams, low appetite, back pain, lower extremities weakness, knee pain and fatigue.

Recommendations: scallions, scallion seeds, lamb, sea cucumber, shrimps, rooster, bitter melon seeds, ginseng, black beans, kidney beans, yams, goji berries, maintaining composure. Tonifying foods are needed, thus many of the remedies include meat, however impotence does not have to be treated with meat.

Remedies:
1. Make lamb stew with daikon radish and Chinese black dates. Drink the broth and eat the lamb.
2. Make cake from black sweet rice, black sesame seeds, black fungus, lotus seeds, walnuts, and black beans. Eat with ½ glass of red wine.
3. Steam rooster with ginger.
4. Dry roast dried shrimps, sea cucumber, and fennel, then grind into a powder. Take one teaspoon three times daily with rice wine.
5. Roast and grind bitter melon seeds. Take one teaspoon three times daily with rice wine.
6. Make tea from walnuts, lotus seeds, pearl barley, Chinese black dates and goji berries. Drink three times daily.
7. Add 50 grams of chopped ginseng to ½ bottle of white liquor (like vodka or gin). Seal bottle, shake bottle daily, and preserve for one month. Drink one shot every night with dinner for at least twenty days.
8. Cook together scallions, shrimp, and egg. Eat with a shot of white liquor.

Avoid: obscene visual stimulation, dairy products, sweets, masturbation, overwork, too much sex

Indigestion

This is a condition of poor digestion due to a weak stomach, lack of digestive enzymes, or eating too fast. This causes a stagnation of food in the stomach, resulting in abdominal fullness or distention, bloating and sometimes diarrhea due to insufficient digestion.

Recommendations: hawthorn berries, papayas, sweet potatoes or yams, daikon radish, black sesame seeds, apples, oranges, parsley. It is important to eat slowly and chew the food properly because digestion begins in the mouth.

Remedies:
1. Dry and age orange peel for about one month. Boil tea and take after meals or simply suck on the peel for indigestion.
2. Eat papaya twice daily, in any form.
3. Eat sweet potato cooked with brown sugar and water. In the last three minutes of cooking this mush, add some rice wine. Eat regularly for two weeks to improve digestion.
4. Blend daikon radish juice and take after meals.
5. Roast black sesame seeds with salt and take with warm water.
6. Eat a leaf of fresh mugwort, or blend into a juice.
7. Drink apple, lemon, or orange juice after meals; or eat an apple after each meal.
8. Consume ½ cup of overdone rice (from bottom of pan) mixed with cardamom, fennel and orange peels.
9. Make tea from sweet rice sprouts and malt.

Avoid: rich foods, fatty foods, tension and stress while eating, reading the newspaper or watching television while eating as this takes energy away from digestion

Kidney Weakness

This common ailment is characterized by weakness and lack of energy. In Chinese medicine, the Kidney system involves much more than just filtering water. It also includes storing the essence of life (sperms and eggs); controlling the bones, bone marrow and the brain (called the *sea of marrow*); growth, maintenance, and reproduction; producing blood; and opening to the ear. The adrenal function is included in the kidney system; thus adrenal exhaustion is Kidney exhaustion. Weakness of the Kidneys often manifests as problems in the back, knees, ears, or reproductive functions. The Kidney is of great importance to health and longevity. Kidney function (and resulting problems) can be divided into Kidney Yang and Kidney Yin.

1. Kidney Yang deficiency

This is characterized by impotence, infertility, coldness, swollen extremities, swollen face, frequent urination, premature ejaculation, diarrhea, low sexual drive, low energy, fatigue, pale face and tongue, low back pain, knee pain or weakness, deafness, ringing in the ears, and a general feeling as though the fire of life is about to be extinguished.

Recommendations: warming foods, chicken, lamb, scallions, sesame seeds, fish, baked tofu, soybeans, walnuts, eggs, lentils, black beans, lotus seeds, a little wine, ginger, cinnamon bark tea

Avoid: cold foods, cold fruits, raw foods

2. Kidney Yin deficiency

In this condition there is not enough water to cool the fire so it manifests as heat symptoms. These may include irritability, insomnia, red cheeks, night sweats, low afternoon fever, damp palms, damp soles of the feet, dry mouth, low back pain, involuntary seminal emissions, ear ringing, red tongue, and blurry vision. Kidney Yin deficiency often occurs in thin people since yin corresponds to substance.

Recommendations: cooling foods, mulberries, apples, peaches, pears, fresh vegetables, mung beans, soybeans, tofu, soy sprouts, chrysanthemum flowers

Avoid: hot foods, spicy foods, smoking, alcohol, stress, and strong emotions

Mastitis

This is an inflammation of the mammary glands, often occurring 3-4 weeks after delivery. It is a very common condition, resulting from an obstructed mammary duct and is accompanied by a bacterial infection. There may be distention of the breast, swelling, redness on the surface, and fever. As the condition progresses, the symptoms may worsen and the patient may have chills, fever, increase in white blood cell count, swollen and painful lymph glands in the armpits, pus and ulceration of breast.

Recommendations: cooling foods such as cabbage, cucumber, dandelion, lettuce, malt, reed root, lotus root, honeysuckle. It is important to keep the affected breast clean.

Remedies:

1. Make tea from malt (sprouted oat), drink three times daily.
2. Externally, take egg white mixed with green onions and apply to the area, changing 2-3 times daily.
3. Make tea from dandelion and honey, drink three times daily for at least five days.
4. Make tea from honeysuckle, mint, and licorice. Drink tea and apply the solids locally.
5. Boil dandelions into tea, condensing to a syrup and add to rice porridge. Eat three times daily for five days.
6. Combine cabbage, lettuce, and dandelions to make a poultice for external application.

Avoid: spicy, stimulating foods, coffee, smoking, alcohol, dairy products (especially if there is pus), breast feeding

Menopause

This is the time when a woman stops menstruating completely, usually occurring between 45 and 53 years of age. It may occur slowly or suddenly. Symptoms may include hot flashes, weakness, depression, emotional instability, anxiety, lack of concentration, irritability, headaches, insomnia, night sweats and dryness.

Recommendations: black beans, sesame seeds, soybeans, walnuts, goji berries, mulberries, yams, licorice, Chinese black dates, lotus seeds, chrysanthemum flowers.

Remedies:
1. Cook black beans with rice into porridge. Eat twice daily.
2. Roast sesame seeds and add to rice porridge for breakfast.
3. Steam chicken with goji berries and yam.
4. Make tea from chrysanthemum and cassia seeds and drink three times daily.
5. Take walnuts, lotus seeds, and sunflower seeds and make a porridge with rice.
6. Stew millet, mulberries, lamb and goji berries.
7. Make tea from licorice, Chinese black dates, and wheat. This will help extreme mood swings and depression.

Avoid: stress, tension, stimulants

Morning Sickness

This is characterized by nausea and vomiting and affects some women during the first few months of pregnancy, usually clearing up after the third month. It occurs particularly in the morning, although in serious cases, it may last all day. Accompanying symptoms may include headache, dizziness, and exhaustion. One should seek treatment right away because this condition will affect nourishment to the fetus.

Recommendations: lentils, grapefruit peel, carp, ginger, orange peel, bamboo shavings, persimmon cap, millet

Remedies:
1. Grind lentils into powder then take two tablespoons with rice porridge, three times daily.
2. Make tea from ginger and grapefruit peel, drink three times daily.
3. Steam carp with ginger and cardamom for thirty minutes. Eat daily for at least one week.
4. Make tea from ginger, orange peels, and a little bit of brown sugar.
5. Make persimmon *cap* tea, drink three times daily.
6. Make fresh scallion juice and fresh ginger juice and add a little sweetener. Take 2-3 teaspoons three times daily.

As soon as the morning sickness stops, discontinue the remedies.

Avoid: overeating, heavy meats

Mouth Sores (Ulcers)

This condition includes herpes simplex, fever blisters and canker sores. It is basically an ulceration on or in the mouth. One may also experience pain, heat sensation, irritability, insomnia, headache, dizziness, palpitations, and bad breath.

Recommendations: mung beans, daikon, carrots, lotus root, persimmon caps, mint, honeysuckle flower

Remedies:
1. Make juice from carrots and lotus root and rinse the mouth 3-4 times a day for at least four days.
2. Take 5-6 persimmon caps and boil tea. When cool, rinse mouth 4-5 times a day.
3. Apply honey to local area to help heal faster.

4. Char eggplant into ashes, powder and mix with honey. Apply to the sores.
5. Boil mung bean soup and eat on an empty stomach.
6. Grind mung beans into powder, mix with honey; apply to area.
7. Rub sea salt on the sores three times a day for two days. Also rinse mouth with salt water.

Avoid: spicy foods, stimulating foods, smoking, stress, alcohol, coffee, chocolate, constipation

Nephritis (Acute)

This is an acute kidney infection. This condition is characterized by some type of infection that precedes the condition, such as laryngitis, tonsillitis, scarlet fever, or mumps. There may be swelling beginning in the face area then spreading throughout the body in about two days, followed by blood in the urine, hypertension, headache, dizziness, fatigue, malaise, low appetite, nausea, vomiting, and scanty urination.

Recommendations: black beans, mung beans, azuki beans, pearl barley, garlic, carp, winter melon, watermelon, watermelon rind, reed root, cornsilk, sweet rice, lotus root, water chestnuts

Remedies:
1. Cook soup with azuki beans, winter melon rind, watermelon rind and cornsilk. Drink at least 3-4 times daily.
2. Make tea from lotus root; drink four large glasses daily.
3. Do a watermelon fast or eat lots of watermelon.
4. Cook soup with carp, azuki beans, winter melon, and green onions. Start with five cups water and cook down to three cups. Drink the soup and sweat.
5. Make tea from cornsilk, cooking for one hour, then strain and cook again until almost dry, then add some fructose powder. Then take one tablespoon three times daily dissolved in warm water.

6. Cook rice porridge with pearl barley, black beans and water chestnuts.
7. Make juice from carrots, celery, cucumbers, and squash.

Avoid: stimulating (sour, spicy, salty) foods, alcohol, caffeine, smoking, overworking, high protein foods

Nephritis (Chronic)

This can result from acute nephritis that is not properly treated, or a low immunity causing kidney infection. The symptoms include swelling, hypertension, hyperprotein urea, fatigue, headache, dizziness, and achiness. If this condition does not get proper treatment, over a long period of time it can cause damage to the kidney, leading to uremia.

Recommendations: ginger, Chinese black dates, sweet rice, soybeans, winter melon, carp, yams, mung beans, black beans

Remedies:
1. Make rice porridge and add ginger, cinnamon, and Chinese black dates. Eat for breakfast and dinner.
2. Remove the internal organs of a duck and stuff it with 4-5 garlic cloves, then cook in soup. Do not add salt. Drink the broth and eat the duck every other day.
3. Cook carp with soybeans, winter melon and green onions into soup. Eat once a day for at least twenty days.
4. Cook rice porridge with yams and eat for breakfast and dinner.
5. Steam together crab, garlic, and white wine. Eat once daily for fifteen days.
6. Boil tea from cornsilk, winter melon rind, watermelon rind, and azuki beans.
7. Crush entire watermelon and rind, and slowly cook to a thick syrup. Take two tablespoons syrup in warm water three times daily.

Avoid: stimulating (sour, spicy, salty) foods, alcohol, caffeine, smoking, overworking, high protein foods

Premenstrual Syndrome (PMS)

PMS is a condition that occurs after ovulation or before menstruation, due to hormonal fluctuations. It may be characterized by abdominal cramps, bloating, backache, headache, tension, irritability, low energy, and mood swings. A healthy woman should have little or no discomfort during this time; however, approximately 70% of American women suffer from these symptoms. This is partially due to the large consumption of cold foods and drinks that can cause the blood to stagnate. In Chinese terminology, PMS is a condition of disharmony in the blood: either stagnant blood, not enough blood, or heat in the blood; and stagnation of Chi. Acupuncture, acupressure, herbs, diet, and Chi gong exercises are all very beneficial for relieving the symptoms and correcting the disharmony.

Recommendations: At least one week prior to the usual onset of PMS symptoms, consume some of the following: ginger, green onions, fennel, orange peel, spinach, walnuts, hawthorn berries, cinnamon, black pepper, Chinese dates, Dang Gui (Angelica sinensis)

Remedies:
1. Make tea from ginger, green onions, fennel, black pepper, and orange peel, boiling for ten minutes. Drink three times daily, starting at least one week before usual onset of PMS symptoms. This is a good remedy for those who feel *cold*.
2. Make spinach soup, boiling for 30 minutes.
3. Make hawthorn berry and cinnamon tea.

Avoid: cold foods, raw foods, excessive consumption of fruit, vinegar, all shellfish, coffee, stimulants, sugar, dairy products, and smoking

Prostate Enlargement

This condition generally affects older men over forty. As the man ages the prostate can become swollen and the urethra and bladder become less elastic. Thus symptoms usually include difficulty urinating or dribbling.

Recommendations: pumpkin seeds, anise, tangerines, cherries, figs, litchis, sunflower seeds, mangos and seaweeds

Remedies:
1. Roast pumpkin seeds or boil into tea and incorporate into the diet, one large handful twice daily.
2. Make tea from rhubarb root, peach kernels, winter melon seeds, pearl barley, azuki beans, and cornsilk; drink three times daily.
3. Boil fig tea.

Avoid: dairy products, rich foods, fatty foods, all stimulants such as alcohol, caffeine, and smoking; stress, tension, sex and eating meat late in the day

Psoriasis

This is a common skin condition, usually genetically inherited, characterized by pink or dull red lesions with silvery scaling. The skin may become very rough and scaly and may temporarily improve, although it is usually a chronic type of condition. When the scaling takes place one can also see reddish dots under the skin, accompanied by various degrees of itching and discomfort. It can affect any part of the body, and is usually worse during the wintertime. In Western medicine there are few treatment options for psoriasis.

Recommendations: Chinese prunes, guava skins, pearl barley, vinegar, garlic, walnuts, cucumber, beet tops, dandelion greens, squash, mung beans

Remedies:
1. Take fifteen peeled and sliced water chestnuts and one cup vinegar (preferably aged rice vinegar), slowly sim-

mer in a non-metal pot for twenty minutes until water chestnuts absorb most of the vinegar. Then mash into a paste and seal in a jar. Spread evenly on a gauze pad and apply to affected area, changing daily if not too serious, three times daily if serious condition. Mild cases should show improvement within five days; serious conditions may take two weeks.

2. Take dried Chinese prunes, remove pits, and simmer into a tea, then condense into syrup. Take two tablespoons in warm water, three times daily.

3. Take peel from guava, char and powder it, mix with sesame oil into a paste and apply twice daily for one week.

4. Apply mashed garlic to the affected area, changing twice daily for one week.

5. Make porridge from lily bulb, gypsum, and rice. Eat once daily for at least ten days.

6. Take mashed walnuts, use cotton to absorb the oil, apply the pulp three times daily.

Avoid: spicy food, stimulating food, alcohol, caffeine, smoking, excessive sun exposure

Seminal Emission (Spermatorrhea)

There are two types of this condition. The first type happens when one has a dream and then ejaculates during sleep, also known as a wet dream. The other type is when one has ejaculation without a dream, either during sleep or during waking hours. One may also have dizziness, back pain, leg pain, weakness, palpitations, shortness of breath, lethargy, or fatigue. These symptoms point to a weakness which if not dealt with can lead to degeneration.

Recommendations: lotus seeds, sea cucumber, yams, dried ginger, scallions, pearl barley, black beans, shrimps, seaweeds, cool showers daily.

Remedies:
1. Steam scallions with shrimp and rice wine. Eat daily for at least fifteen days or until condition improves.
2. Cook soup from sea cucumber, seaweed, and black beans. Walnuts can be added also.
3. Cook sea cucumber with rice porridge and eat for breakfast every morning.
4. Cook pearl barley, black beans, walnuts, and scallions to make a porridge. Eat every morning for breakfast.
5. Make tea from ginseng, Chinese black dates, and lotus seeds. Drink three times daily.

Avoid: spicy foods, stimulating foods, overworking, obscene visual images, masturbation, sleeping on one's back (sleep on the side instead)

Sore throat (Laryngitis)

Sore throat can be caused by various factors including common cold, flu or eating too much spicy food. There may also be mucus, fever and chills, headaches and so on.

Recommendations: carrots, olives, daikon radish, celery, seaweed, licorice, Chinese prunes, cilantro, mint. Drink a lot of water, and gargle with warm salt water

Remedies:
1. Make tea from carrots and olives; drink three times daily for at least one week.
2. Make tea from daikon radish and green apples; drink twice daily.
3. Lightly cook seaweed, preserve with brown sugar for three days. Eat daily for one week.
4. Make tea from cilantro, one tablespoon green tea, and a little salt. Steep for about five minutes.
5. Slowly chew and swallow rock sugar and cilantro.
6. For a dry hot throat, take a spoonful of honey in a glass of warm water and drink.

Avoid: alcohol, smoking, pollution, sleeping with the mouth open, stimulating or spicy foods, fatty foods

Stones (Gallbladder, Kidney, Urinary Tract)

Various combinations of minerals can calcify or crystallize in the gallbladder, kidney, or urinary tract. These can range in size from the size of a grain of sand to two inches in diameter. Gallstones are a combination of bile and minerals and are characterized by pain in the right upper abdomen or pain in the corresponding area of the back and shooting up to the shoulder blade. Gallstones may also cause poor digestion of fats. If the gallstones obstruct the flow of bile, the result may be jaundice. Kidney stones are formed as the kidneys filter excessive minerals in an acid environment which combine with either excessive calcium or wastes in the blood. These are very painful, with the pain being in the kidney area of the lower back or the corresponding area on the front of the abdomen. There may also be painful urination with kidney stones.

Recommendations: cornsilk, water chestnuts, seaweed, beet tops, watermelon, celery, watercress, winter melon, pearl barley, walnuts, watermelon rind, winter melon rind, green tea powder, distilled water

Remedies:
1. Drink watermelon juice.
2. Drink celery, carrot, and water chestnut juice.
3. Drink cornsilk tea for water; 3-5 glasses daily.
4. Drink tea from beet tops, winter melon rind, and watermelon rind.
5. Take two teaspoons ground walnuts in cornsilk tea.
6. Take one teaspoon green tea powder in warm water three times daily.

After consuming any of the above diuretic remedies, do some mild jumping exercise to help break up the stones.

Avoid: spicy foods, fried foods, oily foods, coffee, hard water, spinach, citrus, tomatoes, spinach combined with tofu or dairy products

Tinnitus (Ear Ringing)

This is a common problem that has two major causes. The first is a local problem in which there may be a local obstruction or infection, nerve damage, or drug interference. The second problem stems more from a systemic condition such as coronary heart disease, hypertension, or kidney weakness. Along with ringing in the ears, one may also complain of headaches, irritability, restlessness, dizziness, red face, sore back, vomiting, or nausea.

Recommendations: black sesame seeds, black beans, walnuts, grapes, celery, oyster shells, pearl barley, azuki beans, Chinese black dates, yams, lotus seeds, chestnuts, chrysanthemum. Get plenty of sleep, massage the neck and head area, and try to live in a quiet, peaceful place if possible.

Remedies:
1. Make tea from lotus seeds and chrysanthemums.
2. Make juice from celery and grapes. Drink one cup 2-3 times daily.
3. Cook azuki beans and black beans with rice porridge and eat at least once daily.
4. Boil Chinese black dates, walnuts, and lotus seeds with rice porridge and eat once daily.

Avoid: loud noise, stress, tension, stimulating foods, spicy foods, smoking, alcohol, coffee

Ulcers (Stomach or Duodenum)

Ulcers can occur anywhere along the food pathway, from the mouth to the stomach to the intestines. Ulcers can also occur in the vagina. The most common places for ulcers to occur are the stomach and duodenum (first part of the small intestines).

Ulcers are characterized by burning pain. In the stomach, pain is usually worse on an empty stomach. If the ulcer is further down, there will be pain after meals. There may also be nausea. If the stools are black (digested blood), the ulcer is in the stomach or higher. If stools are red, the ulcer is lower than the stomach. If the red blood is mixed in the stool, the ulcer is in the small intestines. If red blood is on the stool, then the ulcer is in the lower intestines or a result of a hemorrhoid.

Recommendations: potatoes, honey, cabbage, ginger, figs, papayas, squid bone, peanut oil, kale, persimmons, licorice tea

Remedies:
1. For mouth ulcers, apply the ash of charcoaled eggplant.
2. Drink potato juice daily on an empty stomach for at least two weeks.
3. Drink warm kale juice or cabbage juice on an empty stomach to help heal the ulcer.
4. Take two teaspoons peanut oil every morning on an empty stomach to help close the wound.
5. Drink fig juice.
6. Bake squid bone until crisp, powder it and take one teaspoon daily with honey.
7. Take blended papaya and milk or soymilk. Note, this remedy would not be good for a person with a lot of mucus, dampness, or allergies, unless soymilk is substituted for milk.
8. Take two tablespoons steamed honey on an empty stomach in the mornings.
9. Cook ginger (an amount the size of the thumb) with rice and have for breakfast every morning on an empty stomach.
10. Dry and charcoal persimmon and grind into powder; take one tablespoon in a glass of warm water.

Avoid: spicy foods, hot foods, stimulants, shellfish, coffee, smoking, alcohol, fried foods, and stress

Worms

This condition is most common among children. It can manifest in such symptoms as decreased appetite, abdominal pain, nausea, diarrhea or constipation, vomiting, anal itching at night and malnourished appearance. There are many types of worms including roundworms, pinworms, tapeworms, and hookworms.

Recommendations: pumpkin seeds, papaya seeds, coconut, garlic, hawthorn berries, sunflower seeds, Chinese prunes, ginger, vinegar, black pepper, walnut leaf

Remedies:
1. Make tea from ten Chinese prunes, 6 grams black pepper and three slices fresh ginger. Drink two cups, an hour apart in the morning on an empty stomach. Do this every day for one week.
2. Take one tablespoon raw pumpkin seeds and grind to a powder. Mix with warm water and drink. Do this twice daily in the morning an hour apart, every day for one week.
3. Eat two tablespoons sunflower seeds every morning on an empty stomach.
4. Make tea from hawthorn berries and betel nuts and drink two cups in the morning on an empty stomach, one hour apart.
5. Charcoal black pepper, grind to a powder, take ½ teaspoon three times daily with warm water.
6. Make tea from betel nuts and pumpkin seeds. Eat pumpkin seeds then drink the tea and within 4-5 hours expect diarrhea and excretion of the worms.
7. Take the white part of a green onion, make into juice and add 1-2 teaspoons sesame oil. Take twice daily on an empty stomach for three days.
8. Take coconut juice and ½ of a coconut every morning on an empty stomach; wait three hours before eating.
9. Take garlic on an empty stomach every morning.

10. Soak cotton with rice vinegar and plug up anus at night for three days, changing cotton each day. This will attract the worms to the anal area. Or do a rice vinegar enema and hold in all night; do this three days in a row.
11. Mash garlic and mix with Vaseline, apply around anus every night for three days.
12. Mix raw garlic juice and rice vinegar with an equal part water and take on an empty stomach three days in a row.
13. Take one teaspoon ground papaya seeds with warm water every morning on an empty stomach for seven days.

Avoid: unsanitary foods, uncooked meats or fish, raw foods

Section Four

Simple Vegetarian Recipes

Simple Vegetarian Recipes

THESE RECIPES ARE PROVIDED to serve as a guide to those wishing to move away from a heavily meat-based diet. Ideally, meat should comprise no more than 1/10 of the diet. Soy foods such as tofu, tempeh, soymilk and wheat gluten can provide good alternatives to the animal products.

Cooking is an art. To do it well one must be creative, paying attention to how the combinations look as well as how they taste. Always choose foods according to what is seasonally available. Feel free to make substitutions in the recipes with this in mind. Let your taste buds guide you in the appropriate seasonings and combinations of dishes.

Some of the recipes call for *tamari*. This is a naturally aged soy sauce. *Miso* is a salty, aged soybean and grain paste, used for seasoning. Also used for seasoning is *Bragg's Liquid Aminos*, this is a low-salt soy liquid available in health food stores. *Kuzu* and *arrowroot* are thickening agents, similar to cornstarch. *Couscous* is a grain product that comes from the heart of durum wheat and is sweet in flavor.

Many of the recipes use sea vegetables such as *kombu, wakame, nori*, or *hiziki*. Sea vegetables (also known as seaweeds) should be included in the diet regularly for they are an excellent source of nutrients, particularly the minerals. They are also known to alkalinize the body, purify the blood, help dissolve fat and mucous deposits, and neutralize radioactive matter. Seaweeds come in a wide variety of shapes and sizes. The thin sheets called nori can be used to wrap grains or vegetables. Wakame and kombu are good soup additions. Kombu added to beans increases digestibility and decreases cooking time. One of the most flavorful sea vegetables is the red-leafed *dulse*. The adventuresome may wish to try *arame* or *hiziki*; these look like thin black noodles, and are delicious with vegetables or tofu. *Agar flakes* can be used to make a gelatin-like dish called *kanten*.

In general, sea vegetables (except nori) need to be rinsed and soaked prior to using. For soups, washing is sufficient. Dried seaweeds are always available in Asian markets. Many delicious varieties from northern Pacific waters are available in larger health food or grocery stores.

In the recipes that follow, substitutions may be needed to follow a specific remedial diet. For example, a person with candida yeast infection should leave out the tamari and miso (fermented foods) and substitute herb salt or some other seasoning. Someone with a cold type condition may need to add more warming foods to the recipes, such as scallions, garlic, ginger, or pepper. Those with hot type conditions may need to leave out the warming seasonings and so forth.

Imbalances can be well addressed by the addition of therapeutic herbs to the diet. Many of the herbs in the Chinese pharmacopeia were actually recognized as foods prior to their use as medicines. A few of the really delicious ones are lily bulbs, goji berries (Gou Qi Zi, also called lycii berries), Chinese Dioscorea yam, and jujube dates. The typical way of using these *food herbs* would be in soups, stews or grain dishes. The rich colors and textures add a great deal to the dish. For more information on cooking with Chinese herbs and specific recipes read *101 Vegetarian Delights* by Lily Chuang and Cathy McNease, and *Chinese Vegetarian Delights: Sugar and Dairy-Free Cookbook* by Lily Chuang.

The following common abbreviations are used:
t. is teaspoon
T. is tablespoon (3 teaspoons)
c. is cup (8 fluid ounces)

Soups

Sweet Squash and Seaweed Soup
1 stalk celery, diced
1 butternut squash (or other winter squash)
1 small onion or bunch of scallions
Few chopped leaves of Chinese cabbage
1 small piece of wakame seaweed, cut in small pieces
2 T. tamari or Bragg's Liquid Aminos
3 T. garbanzo miso (or other light miso)

Begin with 2 quarts water. Peel and dice the butternut squash and simmer in water, adding the wakame. Add the onion, celery and cabbage. When the vegetables are tender, add the tamari or Bragg's Liquid Aminos and garbanzo miso, which has been dissolved in a small amount of broth. Garnish with a sprig of cilantro. Serves 4.

Summer Vegetable Soup
1 onion
2 carrots
1 clove garlic
1 zucchini
2 tomatoes
1 handful green beans
1 c. fresh corn
1 c. tomato sauce
Herb salt to season
Tamari or Bragg's Liquid Aminos

Chop vegetables into small pieces; add to 2 quarts water. Cook until tender then add 1 c. tomato sauce, heat until warm. Season to taste with herb salt, tamari, or Bragg's Liquid Aminos and garnish with finely chopped cilantro and chives. Serves 4.

Soup Stock

4 six- to eight- inch pieces kombu seaweed
6 Chinese mushrooms
1 carrot
1 stalk celery
1 onion

Add all the above ingredients to 2 quarts water and bring to a boil. Then simmer for 1 hour. Strain and use the liquid for making soups or grains. It will store well in the refrigerator for about a week. Use the vegetables in some dish, perhaps a soup.

Black Bean Soup or Sauce

1 c. black beans
1 four-inch piece kombu
1 small onion, finely chopped
2 garlic cloves
3 T. tamari
1 t. ginger juice
½ red bell pepper
2 T. cilantro

Soak beans overnight. Discard soak water, cover with fresh water and cook beans and kombu for about an hour. You may need to add more water. During the last 20 minutes of cooking, add garlic, onions, and red bell pepper. Mix tamari and ginger juice in at the end. Blend for a creamy sauce to pour over grains or steamed vegetables. Garnish with cilantro. Serves 4.

Beet Soup or Sauce

5-6 carrots
2-3 large beets
2 onions
2-4 stalks celery
3-4 cloves garlic
2 T. miso
2 T. olive oil
1 t. basil, chopped
1 t. oregano, chopped
1 t. umeboshi plum paste

Cook vegetables with 3-4 cups water until tender. Blend vegetables with the cooking liquid. Add the miso, olive oil, basil, oregano, and umeboshi plum paste. Return to flame and simmer for 20 minutes to mix flavors. To make into a sauce, add arrowroot dissolved in ¼ c. water to the mixture and heat until thick and smooth. Serve sauce over noodles or steamed vegetables. Serves 4-6.

Chinese Noodle Soup

8 Chinese mushrooms, soaked with stems removed and sliced
    very thin
6 white mushrooms, sliced very thin
1 red bell pepper, sliced very thin
1 small yellow squash, sliced
1 small piece wakame, sliced into small pieces

Put vegetables into 2 quarts water or vegetable broth and cook
until tender. Then add the following:

3 T. cilantro, chopped
3 green onions, chopped
1 T. tamari
1 t. peanut oil or toasted sesame oil
1 small handful bean threads (mung bean noodles)

Remove from fire and let sit covered for 5 minutes. Serves 4.

Winter Melon Soup

3 qt. vegetable broth
3 c. winter melon, peeled and chopped
2 carrots
2 celery stalks
1 onion
12 Chinese mushrooms, stems removed
6 oz. tofu noodles or finely sliced baked tofu
1 t. chives
1 t peanut oil
1 T. tamari

Cook together until tender, about 25 minutes. Season with
chives, tamari, and peanut oil. Serves 4.

Creamy Split Pea Soup

1 c. green split peas
3 c. water
1 six-inch piece kombu
1 carrot
1 celery stalk
1 small onion
1 t. tamari
½ c. soymilk (or almond milk)
1 T. cilantro
¼ t. paprika
½ t. curry powder
½ t. coriander seed
Pinch nutmeg

Cook peas and kombu until soft. Add the vegetables and cook another 15 minutes. When vegetables are done, put in blender with the tamari, soy milk, cilantro, paprika, curry powder, coriander seed powder, and nutmeg. Serves 4-6.

Grain Dishes

Fancy Rice

1 c. dry brown rice
2 c. water
1 carrot, chopped finely
3 scallions, chopped
¼ red bell pepper, chopped finely

Cook brown rice as usual with water. After about 25 minutes, add the carrot, scallions, and red bell pepper. Cook another 20 minutes or until water is all absorbed. Serves 2.

Nori Burritos

Sheets of nori seaweed
Cooked rice
Carrots, sliced and steamed
Pickled ginger
Sesame seeds, toasted and crushed

Toast sheets of nori seaweed briefly over stovetop flame until it changes color from brown to green (this take about 15 seconds) or use *sushi nori* that has already been toasted. On one end, lay out cooked rice, chopped green onion, steamed carrot slices, pickled ginger, and crushed, toasted sesame seeds. Roll up like a burrito, moistening the edge to make it stick. The edge can be moistened with tamari or Bragg's Liquid Aminos for added flavor.

Vegetable Pie

Crust:
1 c. brown rice
2½ c. water
½ c. couscous
1 c. jicama root, grated
1 t. chives
½ t. basil
¼ t. curry powder
1 t. tamari or Bragg's Liquid Aminos

Filling (finely chopped):
6 oz. tempeh
2 small carrots
1 leek
1 celery stalk
5 Chinese mushrooms, soaked with stems removed

Cook brown rice in water for 30 minutes, then add couscous and cook another 10-15 minutes or until water is absorbed. When done, stir in the jicama, chives, basil, curry powder and tamari. Press into a pie pan and add the filling ingredients.

Steam the pie for 30 minutes. Garnish the top with chopped cilantro. Serves 4-6.

Millet Patties

1 c. millet
2½ c. water
½ t. basil
3 scallions, finely chopped
¼ c. grated carrots
1 T. tamari

Cook millet in water for 30 minutes, or until water is absorbed. Add basil, scallions, carrots and tamari and mix well. Form 2-inch wide patties and put on an oiled cookie sheet. Bake at 325 degrees for 20-30 minutes. They should be crisp on the outside. Serves 4-6.

Stuffed Pumpkin

Cut the top off a small pumpkin; clean out the seeds and strings; save the lid. Fill with the following mixture:

3 c. cooked rice or barley
1 T. toasted sesame seeds, crushed
2-3 stalks celery, chopped
1 onion, finely chopped
1 T. parsley
1 t. thyme
1 t. sage
½ t. rosemary
1 T. tamari

Cover with lid and bake at 350 degrees for 1¼-1½ hours (until fork easily goes into pumpkin).
Serves 4-6.

Simple Couscous Pie

1 c. couscous
¼ c. amaranth or quinoa or millet (presoaked a few hours)
1½ c. boiling water or broth
6 Chinese mushrooms, soaked and sliced
1 c. winter squash, grated or mashed
1 small leek
2 chard leaves
½ red bell pepper
Chopped walnuts

Soak grains in the water 15-30 minutes until soft. Mix with vegetables, all finely chopped. Press into a pie pan and top with chopped walnuts. Steam 40 minutes over medium flame. Serves 6.

Variations:
   1. Substitute 1 c. fresh corn kernels for the red bell pepper.
   2. Substitute 1 c. grated carrot for the squash.
   3. Substitute 1 c. spinach for the chard.

This is an very portable dish and easy to pack for lunch.

Basic Protein Cereal

1 c. brown rice (or ½ barley, ½ brown rice)
1/3 c. soybeans
1 T. sesame or sunflower seeds

Soak above in 3 c. water overnight or in hot water for a few hours. Pour into blender and blend well. Put into a bowl and steam for 1½-2 hours. Serves 4.

Variations:
1. Substitute black or azuki beans for the soybeans.
2. Substitute ½ c. millet for ½ c. brown rice.
3. Substitute walnuts or pecans for the sesame seeds.
4. Season with ginger or cinnamon, or honey or rice syrup, or nut butter.
5. Substitute raw peanuts for the soybeans.

Chestnut Rice

½ c. dried chestnuts
1/3 c. raw peanuts
1 c. brown rice or sweet rice

Soak together the above with 3¾ c. water overnight or in hot water for several hours. Pour into a bowl and steam over low flame for 2 hours, stirring occasionally, until chestnuts are tender. Serves 4.

Variations:
1. Substitute walnuts for the chestnuts
2. Substitute ½ c. barley for ½ c. rice

Simple Grain Dish

1 c. whole grains (brown rice, barley, millet, sweet rice, couscous,
   or a mixture of these)
2 c. water

Preparation:
1. Mix grains and water and steam for 1½-2 hours over a medium flame. Serves 2-4.
2. Use 1 c. grain to 2-2½ c. water to cook grains in pot with lid directly on stove (as opposed to steaming) for 45-50 minutes or until the water is absorbed.

Variations:
1. Add dates or raisins and cinnamon for seasoning.
2. Add steamed peanuts.
3. Add brown rice syrup or maple syrup.

The Fastest Cereal: Couscous

Pour 1 c. boiling water over ¾ c. couscous. Let sit for 5 minutes, covered. Garnish with scallions and cilantro. Serves 2-4.

Variations:
1. Omit the scallions and cilantro and add a grated apple, ¼ c. raisins and a pinch of cinnamon.
2. Add steamed peanuts.
3. Add ½ c. grated carrots and a pinch of ginger.

Steamed Corn Bread

1 c. grated apple (or chopped fresh pineapple)
2 c. coconut milk (or soymilk, or almond milk, or pineapple-coconut juice)
1 medium banana
1/3 c. whole wheat flour
1 c. cornmeal
½ c. oatmeal (or millet flour or brown rice flour)
1/8 c. goji berries or raisins (optional)

Blend the liquid with the banana. Add the rest of the ingredients and mix well. Pour into a pie plate and steam 30 minutes over medium flame. It is done when a chopstick inserted in the center comes out clean. Serves 6.

Variations:
1. Substitute 1 c. grated carrot for the apple or use ½ carrot and ½ apple.
2. Add a pinch of each: cinnamon, ginger, and nutmeg.
3. Add ¼ c. coconut.

Mochi*

Preparation:
1. Soak 2 c. brown or black sweet rice in 2 c. water. Then put in blender, a little at a time. Continue until all is blended.
2. Combine 2 c. powdered brown or black sweet rice and 2 c. water. Mix together well.

Steam for 1½ hours on medium flame, covered. Open and stir well about ½ hour before it is done. Let the rice paste cool.

Use wet hands to handle the rice paste. Form a small ball, flatten between hands, and put a small amount of one of the following fillings in the center: a combination of chopped, cooked Chinese mushrooms, seaweed, baked tofu and seasoning; bean paste (azuki, black, or mung—good in summer); nut butter; or raisins. For a sweeter variety, fill with bean paste and honey or rice syrup. This makes an excellent dessert.

Next, close the patty and form a ball. Roll it over one of the following: sunflower, sesame, or cashew meal, coconut, carob powder, or toasted soybean flour. Serves 4-6.

* This recipe is reprinted courtesy of Lily Chuang from her cookbook, *Chinese Vegetarian Delights: Sugar and Dairy-Free Cookbook* available at www.taostar.com.

Sweet Breakfast Porridge

¾ c. brown rice
¼ c. barley flakes
½ c. raw skinless peanuts
10 Chinese jujube dates
1 slice fresh ginger root

Cook all ingredients with 5 c. water in a crock-pot overnight, or on the stove for 2½-3 hours on low, stirring occasionally. Serves 4.

Bean and Tofu Dishes

Tofu and Mushroom Casserole

2 lb. plain tofu, lightly steamed
12 large Chinese mushrooms, soaked until soft, thinly sliced
2 c. pea pods
1 bunch scallions
2 T. tamari or *Bragg's Liquid Aminos*
3 T. kuzu (or arrowroot or cornstarch)

Slice tofu into 1/2 inch slices and put in bottom of rectangular baking dish. Lightly simmer mushrooms then add pea pods and scallions for last 5 minutes. Put these vegetables on top of the tofu. Use the vegetable cooking water plus enough water to make 3 c. liquid. Add tamari. Dissolve kuzu in a small amount of liquid; add to the rest of the liquid, simmer, stirring often, until the liquid thickens. Pour this gravy on top of the tofu and vegetable mixture. Garnish with crushed, toasted almonds and finely chopped cilantro. Serves 4.

Azuki Bean and Squash Casserole

1 c. azuki beans, soaked overnight
Two 6-8 inch pieces of kombu
1 small butternut squash or other winter squash

Cover beans and kombu with water and simmer about one hour, adding water if needed. Peel and cube the squash and add to the beans. Cook until tender, about ½ hour. Stir in a pinch of sea salt or 1-2 teaspoons tamari. Serves 4.

Clinton's Savory Azuki Beans with Chestnuts

1 c. azuki beans, soaked overnight
¼ c. dried chestnuts, soaked 1 hour
4 six-inch strips kombu seaweed
1 t. tamari or pinch sea salt
1 t. goji berries (optional)

Soak azuki beans overnight; discard soak water. Place kombu in pot then add chestnuts and beans. Cover with 2 inches water and bring to a boil. Simmer 2–3 hours, adding enough water to keep beans covered. Add tamari and the goji berries 10-15 minutes before cooking is done. Serves 4.

Tofu Skins and Mushrooms

12 strips dried tofu skins (available at Asian grocery stores)
6 Chinese mushrooms, thinly sliced, stems removed
8 white mushrooms, sliced
Red bell pepper, sliced
4-6 c. water
2 T. tamari
1-2 T. kuzu (or arrowroot)

Soak the dried tofu skins and Chinese mushrooms in 4-6 cups water and tamari for at least 4 hours. Then tie each strip in a knot, and simmer for 20 minutes. Add the white mushrooms and the red bell pepper and continue to simmer another 10–15 minutes. Pour off the liquid and thicken it with kuzu (do this in a separate pan, heating until thick). Pour the sauce over the tofu and mushroom mixture and serve over steamed greens. Serves 4.

Steamed Peanuts

1 c. raw peanuts
2 c. water

Soak peanuts in water overnight or in hot water for a few hours. Steam using the soaking water for 1½-2 hours over medium flame. This makes a delicious, nutritious addition to cereals, vegetable dishes and grains.

Scrambled Tofu

½ lb. tofu
2 stalks celery
6 white mushrooms
1 tomato
1 t. tamari

Chop vegetables finely. Saute in ¼ c water or 1 T. oil. When almost done, add crumbled tofu. Let heat 5-10 minutes. Season with tamari.

Variations:
1. Substitute one beaten egg for ½ of the tofu.
2. Substitute one small zucchini squash for the mushrooms.

Tofu with Seaweed

1 package baked tofu, sliced or ½ lb. plain tofu, cubed
1 handful hiziki or arame seaweed, soaked in hot water 20-30
  minutes
1 large carrot, diced
½ c. jicama, diced
1 small onion, chopped
4 Chinese mushrooms, presoaked and sliced

Stir-fry carrots, onions, mushrooms and lastly jicama in small amount of water (or mushroom soak water). When almost done, add the tofu and seaweed. Cover and let steam for 5-10 minutes. Season with tamari and toasted sesame oil.

Variations:
1. Substitute wakame or kombu for the hiziki. These need to be presoaked for 1-2 hours.
2. Add diced burdock root (gobo) at the beginning with the carrots.
3. Use white mushrooms instead of the Chinese ones.

Tofu Dressing

½ lb. plain tofu
¼ c. oil
1 T. lemon juice
1 t. honey or rice syrup
1 t. rice or apple cider vinegar
½ t. tamari
1 T. sesame tahini

Blend all the ingredients until creamy. Use on salads, vegetables or sandwiches.

Variations:
1. Add ¼ c. poppy seeds.
2. Add 1½ t. prepared mustard.
3. Add ½ t. basil and ¼ t. garlic powder.
4. Add two whole green onions.

Herbal Dishes

For vegetarians, use vegetable broth instead of chicken broth in the following recipes, and substitute baked tofu for meat or fish. Note: 28 grams = 1 ounce

Basic Herb Soup

1-3 oz. (30-90 grams) herb combination
½–1½ lb. meat or fish (optional)
½ c. grain
¼ c. beans, presoaked (optional)
1-3 c. chopped vegetables
6-8 c. water or broth

Cook herbs, meat, beans, grains and hard vegetables (like carrots, potatoes) about 1 hour, until done. Add soft or leafy vegetables and finish cooking for 15-30 minutes. Season to taste with miso, tamari, soy sauce, rice vinegar or sea salt. The soup could be prepared in a crockpot on high heat for 3-4 hours.

Dang Gui Cornish Hen Stew

1 Cornish hen (or 3 chicken legs)
10 grams Dang Gui (Angelica sinensis)
2 parsnips, chopped
2 carrots, chopped
1 onion, chopped
2 celery stalks, chopped
1 handful wakame or dulse seaweed
8 c. water

Put all ingredients together and simmer for 1 hour. Remove the Cornish hen (or chicken legs). Remove bones, chop meat, and return to the soup. Cook for an additional 15 minutes. Season to taste with miso or soy sauce and chopped cilantro (or parsley). This soup will nourish Chi and blood.

Shan Yao Longevity Stew

10 grams Chinese Yam (Shan Yao)
10 grams goji berries (Gou Qi Zi, also called lycii berries)
10 grams lotus seed (Lian Zi)–presoaked
5 shiitake mushrooms–presoaked
1 onion, chopped
1 carrot or sweet potato, chopped
½ c. white or brown rice
8 c. water (include the shiitake soaking water)

Put all ingredients together and simmer for 1 hour. Season to taste with coriander seed and sea salt. This stew strengthens Spleen and Kidney.

Goji Berry (Gou Qi Zi) Oats

Add a small handful of goji berries (also called lycii berries) and a small handful of almonds (or walnuts) into Scotch oats and cook until soft. Usually 3 parts water to 1 part oats. This will tonify Chi and blood.

Black Bean Stew

Simmer ½ c. black beans with 3 c. water for 1 hour. Then add 6-8 c. chicken broth and the following herbs and vegetables:

1 oz. Shan Yao (Chinese yam)
1 oz. goji berries (Gou Qi Zi)
½ oz. Long Yan Rou (longan fruit)
1 fennel root, chopped
6-7 shiitake mushrooms, soaked and sliced

Simmer the whole dish for 1 hour. Season to taste with sea salt, cumin seeds and brown rice vinegar. This will tonify Chi and blood.

Butternut Mushroom Soup

1 butternut squash, chopped
1 handful wakame seaweed
1 oz. lily bulbs (Bai He)
Enough water to cover vegetables

Cook the above ingredients together until the squash are soft. Remove the butternut squash peel, than blend all ingredients until smooth with the cooking water

In a separate pan sauté in olive oil:

1 purple onion, chopped
2 celery stalks, chopped
12 fresh shiitake mushrooms, sliced

Combine the sautéed ingredients and the blended ones together with the following seasonings:

1 t. basil
1 t. oregano
Sea salt, Bragg's Liquid Aminos or soy sauce, to taste

Sweet and Spicy Pumpkin Soup

1 kabocha squash (Japanese pumpkin)
1 onion, chopped
1 fennel bulb, chopped
1 red bell pepper, chopped

Cook squash in enough water to cover until soft, then blend with the cooking water. Return to pan and add the chopped vegetables and the following presoaked herbs:

1 oz. Chinese yam (Shan Yao)
1 oz. lily bulb (Bai He)
1 oz. goji berries (Gou Qi Zi)
1 oz. longan fruit (Long Yan Rou)

Simmer for 45 minutes. Remove from flame and season with:
1 T. lemon juice
1 t. ginger juice
½ t. cinnamon
½ t. coriander powder
½ t. curry powder
Sea salt or soy sauce to taste

Garnish with chopped cilantro. This soup is both tonifying and calming.

Miscellaneous Recipes

Sesame Seed Garnish

Wash 2 c. whole, brown sesame seeds. Toast in dry skillet, stirring often until seeds can be easily crushed between the fingers. Separately, heat ½ t. sea salt in dry skillet until the chlorine gas is removed (you will smell it). Then mix together sesame seeds and salt and grind in blender or in mortar and pestle. Store in the refrigerator. Use as a garnish for a strong nutty flavor. Salt can be omitted if desired; kelp powder may be substituted for salt.

Basic Vegetable Stir-Fry

Use a variety of vegetables, diced or sliced. Stir-fry in a small amount of water or broth, covered, the slower cooking vegetables and presoaked seaweed first (i.e. carrots, green beans, cauliflower, nori, kombu, etc.), then add the faster cooking vegetables (i.e. jicama, zucchini, broccoli, etc.) When the last vegetables go in, you can add tofu or gluten pieces.

When the vegetables and seaweed are cooked, season to taste with oil, soy sauce (or Bragg's Liquid Aminos), herb salt, or your favorite cooking herbs. Basil and cilantro are particularly good with vegetables.

Variations:
1. Add steamed peanuts or almonds.
2. Add one garlic clove at the beginning.
3. Add finely grated ginger toward the end of the cooking.
4. Add chopped green onions at the end.
5. Add Chinese mushrooms (presoaked) at the beginning.

Almond Nut Stir-Fry

1 small yam
1 small head cauliflower
1 leek or onion
2 summer squash
1 handful green beans
¼ lb. white mushrooms
½–¾ c. almonds
½ t. toasted sesame oil
1 T. arrowroot (or cornstarch)

Chop vegetables into small pieces. Put in skillet with about ¼ inch water. Cover and steam until vegetables are tender. Pour out any remaining water into a bowl. Add arrowroot and stir until dissolved; pour back into vegetables and heat briefly until liquid thickens. Stir in almonds and toasted sesame oil. Garnish with toasted sesame seeds. Serves 2-4.

Stir-Fry Over Noodles

2 c. broccoli, chopped
1 red bell pepper, sliced
2 garlic cloves
1 zucchini, diced
2 leeks, chopped
1 carrot, diced
5 white mushrooms, sliced
1 T. peanut oil
¼ c. water or broth

Heat peanut oil and saute the garlic and leeks. Add the mushrooms, carrots, broccoli, and water or broth. Cover and cook 5 minutes. Lastly, add the zucchini and red bell pepper and cook another 5 minutes. Season to taste with basil, cilantro, and tamari. Serve over whole wheat or tofu noodles. Serves 2-4.

Almond Milk

1 c. raw almonds
2 c. water
½ t. vanilla or almond extract
2 T. honey or maple syrup
Pinch cinnamon

Soak almonds for at least 4 hours. Grind in blender with water, strain and put the solids back in the blender and repeat the process two more times. Combining all of the strained milk there should be a total of 6 cups. Put some of the liquid back in the blender with the vanilla, honey and cinnamon. Blend and mix back into the other liquid. Store in the refrigerator and use within a few days. Almond milk can also be sweetened by grinding in 5-6 dates or a small handful of raisins. This same procedure can be used to make other nut milks like cashew or sesame milk.

Soybean Milk

Soak soybeans at least 8 hours, or as long as three days in the refrigerator. Blend soaked beans with 3 c. water, then strain through a cloth, squeezing out the milk. Put the pulp back in the blender with more water and repeat the process until you have 1½ quarts of soymilk. Bring to a boil and simmer for 15-20 minutes, stirring often to prevent sticking and boiling over. Soymilk can be used plain, mixed with carob powder and rice syrup, or blended with fruits such as papaya or banana (cool soymilk before mixing with fruit).

Protein Pudding

3 c. soymilk
1/3 c. rice syrup (or maple syrup)
1 bar agar seaweed

Rinse agar, then mix with soymilk. Cook together until agar is dissolved. Stir in syrup. Pour into dishes and let firm.

Variations:
1. Add ½ c. raisins or chopped dates.
2. Add ½ c. pecans, sunflower seeds, walnuts, or cashews.
3. Flavor with ½ t. vanilla or 3 T. carob powder.
4. Substitute almond milk for the soymilk and garnish the top with ¼ c. almonds when almost firm.

Pecan Pudding

2 c. soymilk
½ c. pecans or walnuts
¼–1/3 c. maple or brown rice syrup
3 T. arrowroot (or kudzu or sweet rice flour)
2 T. carob powder

Blend all ingredients well. Heat over low flame until thickened, stirring constantly. Serve warm.

Wheat Gluten (Wheat Meat)

2½ lbs. gluten flour (or unbleached white flour or whole wheat
  flour)
1 qt. water
Tamari to season

Mix flour and water until it forms a stiff dough. Let sit one
hour. Then cover with water and knead with both hands.
Pour off the starchy white water and repeat the process until
the water is clear. This will take many washings and much
kneading. For tender gluten, cover the finished gluten with
water and let stand for 1-2 days before using. To cook, drop
small pieces into boiling water for 30 minutes. Remove from
water and season with tamari. Gluten can also be marinated
before or after cooking. Tamari, ginger, garlic, and onions make
a good marinade. Gluten can be used whenever a "meaty"
textured food is desired.

Basic Tomato Sauce

3 c. chopped tomatoes
1 bell pepper, chopped
1 garlic clove
1 small onion, chopped
2 T. fresh basil (or ½ t. dried)
½ t. oregano
1 t. onion powder
1½ T. tamari
2 T. arrowroot (or kudzu or cornstarch)

Cook the tomatoes, bell pepper, garlic and onion until tender.
Then put in blender with the basil, oregano, onion powder and
tamari. Return to pan when well blended. Mix arrowroot with
a small amount of water. Add to the tomato mixture, and heat
stirring often until thick.

Variations for Basic Tomato Sauce:
1. Add ½ c. sautéed white mushrooms.
2. Add ½ c. zucchini
3. Serve over noodles or steamed spaghetti squash.

Simple Oil and Vinegar Dressing

½ c. oil
½ c. vinegar, rice or apple cider
Lemon juice (optional)
1 T. tamari or Bragg's Liquid Aminos (optional)
¼ t. garlic or onion powder

Blend the oil and vinegar by whisk, shaker or blender. You may add the optional ingredients. For an Italian dressing, add ½ t. oregano and ½ t. basil to the oil and vinegar mixture.

Coriander Vinaigrette

2 T. coriander seeds
½ c. olive oil
¼ c. brown rice vinegar
½ bunch cilantro, roughly chopped
1 T. shallots or chives, chopped
Salt and pepper to taste

Blend together until smooth. Serve over mixed greens or grains.

Lemon Vinaigrette

1 clove garlic
½ lemon, whole with seeds removed
½ c. chopped sweet onion
½ c. lemon juice
1½ t. Dijon mustard
½ c. red wine vinegar
½ t. honey
½ t. pepper
½ t. salt
2 c. olive oil

Blend together until smooth. Serve over dark leafy greens for a Liver benefiting effect.

Pecan Dressing

½ c. sesame oil
½ c. toasted pecans
½ c. coconut milk
3 T. lemon juice
2 T. honey
Salt to taste

Blend the above ingredients together and serve over the following cole slaw:

½ c. each: finely shredded cabbage, fennel and carrots
1/3 c. chopped crystallized ginger
1 T. coriander or fennel seeds
¾ c. cilantro, chopped

Sprouts

Sprouts are easy to grow and very nutritious. The nutritional value of sprouts is increased manifold over the unsprouted seeds.

Rainbow Mix

This is a blend of azuki beans, mung beans and lentils. Soak seeds (together or separately) overnight. Pour off the soak water and rinse twice daily. A jar with a screen on top is very handy for growing sprouts. Store in a warm, dark place for 3-5 days remembering to rinse twice daily. At the end of the growth period, put in sunlight for 30-60 minutes for the leaves to produce chlorophyll. These can be eaten raw or lightly sautéed. Whole peas or whole wheat may also be added to this mix.

Light Mix

This blend is alfalfa seeds, red clover seeds and daikon radish seeds (optional). Sprout these in the same fashion as above. These sprouts can be eaten raw as a garnish in salads and sandwiches.

Sandwich Fillings

These fillings can be used with any whole grain bread or pita (pocket) breads or rolled inside whole wheat tortillas (chapatis).

Rainbow Sprouts

Lightly saute the following in water or oil: mung, azuki and lentil sprouts, grated carrots, shredded red cabbage, soaked hiziki seaweed and grated ginger.

Garbanzo Spread

Cook garbanzo beans until soft. Mash and mix with sesame tahini, lemon juice, garlic powder and a pinch of salt. Garnish with alfalfa/clover sprouts and tomato slices.

Nut Butter

Blend almond butter, sesame butter, or cashew butter, grated carrots, green onions and cilantro.

Soy Burger

Combine cooked soy and garbanzo beans, grated carrots, sliced mushrooms, and enough cornstarch or arrowroot or flour to hold together. Steam for 15-20 minutes over medium flame.

Sweet Treat

Combine almond butter, rice syrup, grated apple and a pinch of ginger or cinnamon.

Eggplant Spread

Steam eggplant until soft. Mash and mix with sesame tahini, garlic and lemon juice.

Colorful Sandwich

Steam beets and carrots. Mash and mix with sautéed, finely chopped tofu, cabbage, and celery.

Congee Recipes

A *congee* (also known as *jook*, porridge or gruel) is a soupy grain dish typically eaten for breakfast. It may be used for other meals by those who are weak or chronically ill. Congees are highly digestible, easily assimilated, and good for people with weak digestion, fatigue, or poor appetite and those who are convalescing from surgery or illness.

Traditionally cooked with rice or millet, congees can be cooked with other grains, or a combination of grains, including barley, cornmeal, and quinoa. The basic recipe can be modified with the addition of therapeutic foods, medicinal herbs, and spices.

Basic Congee Recipe
1 c. rice (white, brown, sweet, basmati)
5-10 c. water (depending on how thick or thin you want the dish to be)

Cook for about 4-6 hours on a low flame or overnight in a crock pot. The finished congee can be mildly seasoned with sea salt, miso or honey.

Congee variations to be added at the beginning of the cooking process:

¼ c. mung beans to clear heat and toxins
¼ c. aduki beans
¼ c. Job's tears or pearled barley (Yi Yi Ren) to promote urination, reduce damp and heat
2 chopped celery stalks to clear heat, reduce hypertension
1 chopped carrot to promote digestion and strengthen the Lung
1 t. fennel seeds or coriander seed to relieve gas and bloating
5 pitted Chinese dates (Da Zao) and 3 slices fresh ginger to harmonize the Stomach and relieve nausea or vomiting
¼ c. goji berries (Gou Qi Zi) to benefit the eyes and nourish blood and Yin
10 grams astragalus (Huang Qi), 10 grams Chinese yam (Shan Yao) and 5 shiitake mushrooms to benefit the immune system (remove the astragalus at the end of cooking as it remains woody)
¼ c. dried seaweed such as wakame, nori or dulse to reduce yellow phlegm
2 t. turmeric powder to activate the blood and relieve pain
½ c. chopped walnuts, almonds, pine nuts or sesame seed to promote a bowel movement
1 chopped pear
¼ c. chopped almonds to descend the Lung chi and stop cough

Congee variations to be added at the end of the cooking, the last 10-15 minutes:

¼ c. chopped mint to promote sweat and relieve fever and sore throat
¼ c. chopped parsley to promote digestion and relieve food stagnation, bloating and indigestion
¼ c. chopped scallions and 6 slices of fresh ginger to relieve chills and nasal congestion

Section Five

Sample Meal Plans

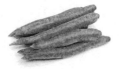

Sample Meal Plans

Our meal plans are intended to provide some direction in nutritional meal planning. They are not meant to be a rigid regimen, rather a framework within which to plan your meals. Feel free to make substitutions to suit your individual needs. If your diet includes fish and meat, they may be substituted for tofu or other soy products for up to 10% of your diet. If your diet includes eggs or dairy products, those too can be substituted as protein sources.

In general, each meal will be constructed around a grain food with fresh vegetables and fruits. As a vegetarian, it is important to eat a variety of bean foods also to provide a more balanced protein than grain alone. Examples are soybean milk over oatmeal, lentils and rice, or black bean soup with corn bread. Dairy products, eggs, nuts and seeds are also used to complement grain or bean protein.

Breakfast should sustain us through the first portion of our productive day, so don't skimp on it. Lunch is usually lighter because of the typical time frame within which we have to eat at midday, although this is an ideal time for the biggest meal of the day. Dinnertime is usually more leisurely, and allows for more creativity in the kitchen. Try not to overeat before bedtime.

In the spring/summer, we tend to eat lighter and include more fresh fruits and cooling foods. Moister foods will be needed during the hot and dry season. Fall/winter meals need to provide extra fuel to sustain our energy and keep us warm. Thus we will need to eat more baked and warming foods during the cold season.

Spring/Summer Meals

Monday

BREAKFAST
- Cream of rice or wheat with raisins and cinnamon
- Steamed apple

LUNCH
- Winter melon soup with tofu*
- Rice cake with nut butter

DINNER
- Stir-fried vegetables with tofu and gluten*
- Brown rice*

Tuesday

BREAKFAST
- Scrambled tofu with tomato and zucchini
- Brown rice with pecans

LUNCH
- Chinese noodle soup*
- Couscous with steamed peanuts*
- Papaya slices

DINNER
- Fancy rice*
- Brown rice*

Please note: Those dishes that are marked with an asterisk (*) are listed in the recipe section. Detailed preparation instructions are included.

Wednesday

BREAKFAST
- Apple/banana or carrot corn bread*
- Soybean milk*

LUNCH
- Fruit salad with soy yogurt and almonds
- Brown rice drink (amasake)

DINNER
- Tomato-mushroom sauce over whole-wheat noodles and tempeh cubes*
- Steamed broccoli

Thursday

BREAKFAST
- Couscous with grated apples and raisins*
- Almond milk*

LUNCH
- Nori rolls with rice, steamed carrots and stir-fry cilantro*
- Brown rice drink (amasake)

DINNER
- Vegetable tofu stir-fry*
- Mochi rice balls*

Friday

BREAKFAST
- Steamed pineapple corn bread*
- Almond pudding*

LUNCH
- Pita bread with rainbow sprouts and carrots*
- Green salad with tofu dressing*

DINNER
- Tofu skins and mushrooms*
- Brown rice*
- Steamed eggplant

Saturday

BREAKFAST
- Simple cereal with dates, raisins, and sunflower seeds

LUNCH
- Summer vegetable soup*
- Chapatis with avocado and sprouts

DINNER
- Couscous-corn pie*
- Green salad with sesame garnish*

Sunday

BREAKFAST
- Scrambled tofu with egg*
- Couscous pie*
- Soybean milk*

LUNCH
- Garbonzo spread on whole-wheat bread*
- Apple slices

DINNER
- Vegetable stir-fry*
- Protein cereal with peanuts and pecans*

Fall/Winter Meals

Monday

BREAKFAST

- Basic protein cereal with azuki or black beans
- Steamed tofu with ginger, soy sauce, and nut meal

LUNCH

- Stir-fry vegetables with tofu and seaweed*
- Simple grain dish*

DINNER

- Tofu skins with Chinese mushrooms*
- Rice/barley/couscous*
- Steamed broccoli

Tuesday

BREAKFAST

- Simple cereal with dates, raisins, and peanuts*
- Steamed corn bread with sesame butter and rice syrup*

LUNCH

- Soyburger sandwich*
- Vegetable soup

DINNER

- Couscous-corn pie*
- Azuki beans and chestnuts*
- Steamed spinach

Wednesday

BREAKFAST
- Simple cereal with ginger, scallions, and miso*
- Steamed broccoli and green beans
- Soy milk*

LUNCH
- Nori burritos*
- Black bean soup*

DINNER
- Tofu-mushroom casserole*
- Stuffed pumpkin*
- Pecan pudding*

Thursday

BREAKFAST
- Steamed corn bread with black bean spread and sliced banana*
- Soy milk with carob*

LUNCH
- Vegetable pie*
- Steamed greens

DINNER
- Cashew stir-fry*
- Millet and rice*
- Protein pudding*

Friday

BREAKFAST
- Steamed corn, beets, and spinach
- Pita bread sandwiches with mochi*
- Cinnamon soy milk*

LUNCH
- Stir-fry vegetables over noodles*
- Sweet squash and seaweed soup*

DINNER
- Azuki bean and squash casserole*
- Sweet brown rice and couscous*
- Cauliflower

Saturday

BREAKFAST
- Simple cereal with tempeh, mushrooms, and celery*
- Steamed apples

LUNCH
- Creamy split pea soup*
- Millet patties*

DINNER
- Beet sauce over noodles*
- Tofu and Chinese mushrooms*

Sunday

BREAKFAST
- Chestnut rice with peanuts*
- Steamed carrots

LUNCH
- Chapatis with rainbow sprouts and carrots*
- Steamed yam

DINNER
- Black bean over rice*
- Vegetable stir-fry*

Section Six

Appendix

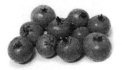

Chart 1: Energetic Properties of Foods
Vegetables

Cold	Cool	Neutral	Warm	Hot
Chinese cabbage	Alfalfa sprouts	Chard	Bell pepper	Garlic
Mung bean sprouts	Asparagus	Jerusalem artichoke	Chinese chives	Scallions
Seaweed	Bamboo shoots	Lettuce	Ganoderma	
Snow peas	Beets	Shitake mushrooms	mushrooms	
Water chestnut	Bok choy	Sweet potato	Green beans	
White mushrooms	Broccoli	Taro root	Kale	
	Burdock root	Yam	Leek	
	Button mushrooms		Mustard Green	
	Cabbage		Onion	
	Carrot		Parsley	
	Cauliflower		Parsnip	
	Celery			
	Cilantro			
	Collards			
	Corn			
	Cucumber			
	Daikon radish			
	Dandelion greens			
	Eggplant			
	Endive lettuce			
	Lotus root			
	Potato			
	Pumpkin			
	Romaine lettuce			
	Soybean sprouts			
	Spinach			
	Summer squash			
	Turnip			
	Watercress			
	Winter melon			
	Winter squash			
	Zucchini			

Energetic Properties of Foods (continued)

Fruits

Cold	Cool	Neutral	Warm	Hot
Banana	Apple	Chinese date	Blueberry	Hawthorn berry
Cantaloupe	Apricot	Coconut milk	Cherry	Litchi (lychee)
Grapefruit	Avocado	Goji berry	Chinese prune	Papaya
Mulberry	Cranberry	Loquat	Coconut	Pineapple
Pear	Fig	Mango	Dried papaya	Plum
Pear-apple	Lemon	Olive	Grape	Raspberry
Watermelon	Limes			Tangerine
	Orange			
	Peach			
	Persimmon			
	Strawberry			
	Tomato			

Grains

Cold	Cool	Neutral	Warm	Hot
	Barley	Buckwheat	Amaranth	
	Kamut	Brown rice	Oats	
	Millet	Corn meal	Quinoa	
	Pearl barley	Rice bran	Spelt	
	White rice	Rye	Sweet rice	
	Wheat		Wheat bran	
			Wheat germ	

Seeds and Beans

Cold	Cool	Neutral	Warm	Hot
Pumpkin seeds	Mung beans	Almond	Black bean	Navy bean
	Lima beans	Azuki bean	Brown sesame seed	Pecan
	Soybeans	Black sesame seed	Cashew	Pine nut
	Tofu	Filbert	Chestnut	Pinto bean
	Winter melon seeds	Kidney bean	Garbonzo bean	Walnut
		Lotus seed	Lentil	
		Peanut		
		Pea		
		Sunflower seed		

Animal Products

Cold	Cool	Neutral	Warm	Hot
Pork	Chicken egg	Dairy products	Beef	Lamb
	Clam	Duck	Chicken	
	Crab	Fish (ocean)	Fish (freshwater)	Shrimp
		Gelatin	Goat's milk	Turkey
		Oyster	Quail egg	

217

Energetic Properties of Foods (continued)

Herbs

Cold	Cool	Neutral	Warm	Hot
Bamboo shavings	American ginseng	Chinese yam	Anise seed	Fresh ginger	Black pepper
Cassia seeds	Cilantro	Licorice root	Basil	Hawthorn berry	Cinnamon bark
Chinese cucumber	Corn silk	Loquat leaf	Cardamom seed	Longan fruit	Dry ginger
Chrysanthemum	Kudzu (pueraria root)	Lycii (goji) berry	Carob pod	Mugwort	
Goldenseal root	Mint leaf	Poria mushroom	Citrus peel	Oriental ginseng	
Gypsum		Peach kernel	Clove	Squid bone	
Honeysuckle flower		Persimmon cap	Coriander seed		
Lily bulb			Dang gui		
Mother of pearl shell			Fennel seed		
Motherwort leaf					
Mulberry leaf					
Oyster shell					
Reed root					

Miscellaneous

Cold	Cool	Neutral	Warm	Hot
Salt	Tea (green)	Barley malt	Brown sugar	
Vitamin C	Spirulina	Rice malt	Coffee	
White sugar	Chlorella	Black fungus	Molasses	
		Honey	Rice vinegar	
		White fungus	Wine	

218

Chart 2: Five Elements Correspondences

	Wood	Fire	Earth	Metal	Water
Organ	Liver, Gall bladder	Heart, Small Intestine, Pericardium, Sanjiao	Spleen, Stomach Pancreas	Lungs, Large intestine	Kidneys Bladder
Flavor	Sour	Bitter	Sweet	Pungent	Salty
Sense	Sight/eyes	Taste/tongue	Touch/skin	Smell/nose	Hearing/ears
Color	Green	Red	Yellow	White	Black
Emotion	Anger	Joy (mania)	Worry	Sadness	Fear
Voice	Shouting	Laughter	Singing	Crying	Groaning
Physical manifestation	Muscles and tendons	Blood vessels	Flesh	Skin and body hair	Bone
Mode of action	Twitching	Itching	Hiccuping	Coughing	Shivering
Internal energy	Hun Chi (psychic Chi)	Shen Chi (directing Chi)	Yuan Chi (primal Chi)	Po Chi (physical Chi)	Ching Chi (creative Chi)
Body fluid	Bile and tears	Blood and sweat	Saliva	Jin (mucous secretions)	Sexual fluids
Climate	Wind	Heat	Humidity	Dryness	Cold
Season	Spring	Summer	Late summer and between seasons	Autumn	Winter

219

Five Elements Correspondences *(continued)*

	Wood	Fire	Earth	Metal	Water
Orientation	East	South	Center	West	North
Development	Birth	Growth	Maturity	Harvest	Storage
Negative drive	Hostility	Greed	Ambition	Stubbornness	Desire
Corrupting influence	Competition	Sex	Mind	Money	Alcohol
Attributes of mind	Rationality	Spirituality	Tranquility	Sentimentality	Desire
Moral trait	Benevolence	Humility	Trustfulness	Rectitude	Wisdom

Chart 3: Five Energetic Transformations

The Creation Cycle

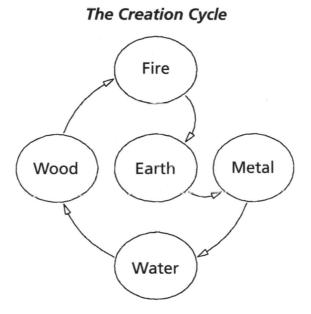

The Control Cycle

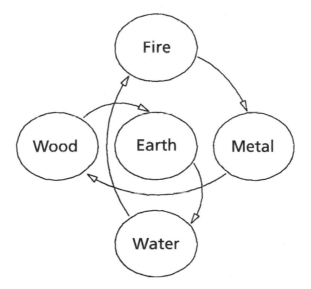

Chart 4: Translations of Food & Herb Names

Name	Pin Yin	Latin	Other
alismatis root	ze xie	Rhizoma Alismatis	
abalone shell	shi jue ming	Concha Haliotidis	
American ginseng	xi yang shen	Radix Panacis Quinquefolii	
apricot kernels	xing ren	Semen Armeniacae Amarum	
astragalus	huang qi	Radix Astragali	
bamboo shavings	zhu ru	Caulis Bambusae in Taenia	`
betel nut	bing lang	Semen Arecae	
black fungus	hei mu er	Auricularia Auricula	wood ears
black sesame seed	hei zhi ma	Semen Sesami Nigrum	
burdock root	niu bang gen	Radix Arctii	gobo
cardamom seed	bai dou kou	Fructus Amomi Rotundus	
	sha ren	Fructus Amomi Villosum	
cassia seeds	jue ming zi	Semen Cassiae	
chicken gizzard	ji nei jin	Endothelium Corneum Gigeriae Galli	
Chinese cucumber	tian hua fen	Radix Trichosanthis	
Chinese date	da zao	Fructus Jujubae	
Chinese date (black)	hei zao	Fructus Jujubae	
Chinese date (red)	hong zao	Fructus Jujubae	
Chinese prune	wu mei	Fructus Mume	
Chinese yam	shan yao	Rhizoma Dioscoreae	
chrysanthemum	ju hua	Flos Chrysanthmi	
citrus peel	chen pi	Pericarpium Citri Reticulatae	
cinnamon bark	rou gui	Cortex Cinnamomi	
clematis	wei ling xian	Radix Clematidis	
cloves	ding xiang	Flos Caryophylli	
cornsilk	yu mi xu	Stigma Maydis	
dandelion	pu gong ying	Herba Taraxaci	
dang gui	dang gui	Radix Angelica Sinensis	
fennel seed	xiao hui xiang	Fructus Foeniculi	
fritillaria bulb	chuan bei mu	Bulbus Fritillariae Cirrhosae	
ganoderma mushroom	ling zhi	Ganoderma	reishi
ginger root (fresh)	sheng jiang	Rhizoma Zingiberis	
ginger root (dried)	gan jiang	Rhizoma Zingiberis	
ginkgo nut	bai guo	Semen Ginkgo	

Translations of Food & Herb Names *(continued)*

Name	Pin Yin	Latin	Other
goji berry	gou qi zi	Fructus Lycii	lycii
gypsum	shi gao	Gypsum Fibrosum	
hawthorn berry	shan zha	Fructus Crataegi	
honeysuckle	jin yin hua	Flos Lonicerae	
kudzu	ge gen	Radix Puerariae	kuzu
licorice	gan cao	Radix Glycyrrhizae	
ling zhi mushroom (See ganoderma mushroom)			
litchi kernel	li zhi he	Semen Litchi	
loquat leaf	pi pa ye	Folium Eriobotryae	
lotus root	lian gen	Rhizoma Nelumbinis	
lotus seed	lian zi	Semen Nelumbinis	
lychee	li zhi	Litchi chinensis	litchi
lycii berry	gou qi zi	Fructus Lycii	goji
lily bulb	bai he	Bulbus Lilii	
longan fruit	long yan rou	Arillus Longan	
malt syrup	yi tang	Saccharum Granorum	barley malt
mother of pearl shell	zhen zhu mu	Concha Margaritae	
motherwort leaf	yi mu cao	Folium Leonuri	
mulberry	sang shen	Fructus Mori	
mugwort	ai ye	Folium Artemisiae argyi	
mung bean	lu dou	Semen Phaseoli radiati	
Oriental ginseng	ren shen	Radix Ginseng	
oyster shell	mu li	Concha Ostreae	
peach kernel	tao ren	Semen Persicae	
pearl barley	yi yi ren	Semen Coicis	coix Job's tears
persimmon cap	shi di	Calyx Kaki	
poria mushroom	fu ling/fu shen	Poria	
prunes (unripe)	wu mei	Fructus Mume	
pumpkin seed	nan gua zi	Semen Cucurbitae	
raspberry	fu pen zi	Fructus Rubi	
reed root	lu gen	Rhizoma Phragmitis	
squid bone	hai piao xiao	Endoconcha Sepiae	
walnut	hu tao ren	Semen Juglandis	
white fungus	bai mu er; yi er	Tremella	silver ears
winter melon seed	dong gua ren	Semen Benincasae	

Glossary

Astringent – substance that has a constricting action or causes contraction of orifices. Examples of astringent action are to stop sweating or stop diarrhea.

Arteriosclerosis – hardening of the arteries, usually due to aging or high consumption of fatty foods over a long period of time.

Ascites – accumulation of fluids in the abdomen, usually due to cirrhosis of the liver.

Cap – calyx; the sepals of a flower. A persimmon cap is the green papery calyx at the stem end of the orange fruit.

Carminative – substance that promotes normal flow of energy and removes obstructions; substance that relieves gas from the gastrointestinal tract.

Chi (qi) – energy or life force; an entity that denotes the functional aspect of the body in Chinese Medicine.

Chi gong (qi gong) – a set of breathing exercises for strengthening and balancing the energy (Chi), relaxing the mind, and for the purpose of maintaining health and curing disease.

Clears heat – to remove or neutralize pathogenic heat from the body; to soothe a hot, feverish condition with cooling foods or herbs.

Colitis – inflammation of the colon.

Cold type condition – a condition caused by cold, one of the six pathogenic factors in the environment, or simply the result of insufficient fire (Yang) in the body. It is benefited by warming foods and herbs, and application of warmth (i.e. heating pad) and is aggravated by cold.

Cold type person – one who frequently tends to feel cold, be pale-complexioned, lack energy, tend toward loose stools.

Conjunctivitis – inflammation and infection of the mucous membranes of the eyelids as a result of too much heat in the body, specifically in the Liver, according to Chinese Medicine.

Consolidate (the lungs) – to strengthen the lungs in conditions of chronic cough, asthma and shortness of breath.

Cooling food – a food that has a counteracting effect to heat in the body, i.e., elicits a cooling response from the body; food of a Yin nature, food that lowers metabolism.

Dampness – one of the external causes of disease that disturbs the normal flow of energy and particularly the digestive functioning of the Spleen and Stomach, characterized by heaviness, stagnation, and turbidity; fluid accumulation due to impaired water metabolism.

Deficiency – condition of weakness or lack of either energy or substance due to illness or improper lifestyle, diet, or mental attitude.

Descend – to move energy in a downward direction in the body.

Diaphoretic – a substance that induces perspiration in order to expel pathogenic factors and toxins.

Disharmony – imbalance or disease or lack of healthy function.

Diuresis – a process that promotes smooth urination and reduces edema.

Diuretic – a food or herb that promotes urination in order to relieve swelling or discomfort in urination.

Dryness – one of the six pathogenic factors in the environment. Disorders with dryness are associated with thirst, dry mouth and throat, fever, constipation, scanty concentrated urine, dry cough and emaciation. This can also be due to internal imbalances in the body.

Dysentery – extreme diarrhea and tenesmus due to bacterial or viral infection.

Dysuria – painful or difficult urination.

Edema – abnormal accumulation of fluids in the body; swelling.

Essence ("Jing") – the source of life, found in eggs, sperm, marrow, and the brain and stored in the Kidneys; provides for growth, development and reproduction throughout one's entire lifetime.

Five Element Theory – an ancient philosophical concept to explain the phenomena of energy transformation and the composition and relationships of the natural world and the human body. A further refinement of the concept of opposites (Yin and Yang) into four degrees, the fifth being the center or balance. For a more thorough understanding of the Five Element Theory, please refer to *Tao, The Subtle Universal Law* by Hua-Ching Ni.

Gastritis – inflammation of the stomach.

Gruel (congee or porridge) – grain that has been cooked with extra water and cooking time to the point of being *soupy*.

Harmonize – restore general balance; to bring together into smooth functioning.

Hot type condition – a condition that is usually caused by heat, one of the six pathogenic factors in the environment, or a lack of water (Yin) to counterbalance the fire (Yang) in the body. It is benefited by cooling foods and treatment, and aggravated by heat. This is usually an acute, excess condition, i.e., infections, fevers and boils.

Hot type person – one who frequently tends to feel hot, sweat freely, be red in face or tongue, have an excess of energy, be thirsty.

Hypertension – high blood pressure.

Lactostasis – hampered milk production or secretion due to physical or functional obstruction.

Leukorrhea – white or yellow mucous discharge from the cervix or the vagina.

Liver heat (or fire) rising – a condition in which an excessive amount of heat in the Liver rises to the upper part of the body causing red painful eyes, flushed cheeks, headache, fits of anger, emotional instability, dizziness, ringing in the ears and insomnia.

Neurasthenia – nervous exhaustion characterized by fatigue, weakness, headache, sweating, polyuria, tinnitus, dizziness, fear, photophobia and insomnia.

Pathogen – a microorganism or substance capable of producing a disease. In Chinese Medicine, it refers to anything that may cause imbalance within the body including environmental factors (wind, cold, heat, dampness, dryness, summer heat) and emotions.

Qi *(see Chi)*

Qi gong *(see chi gong)*

Rebellious Chi – energy that moves upwardly when it normally should be going down, i.e. coughing, vomiting and hiccuping.

Shen – spirit.

Stagnancy – a sluggishness or impeded circulation of blood, Chi, or body fluids.

Summer heat – one of the external causes of disease characterized by irritability, fever, headache, thirst, restlessness and sweating

Tai Chi Chuan – an ancient Chinese exercise for harmonizing the mind, body and spirit. The connected movements somewhat resemble a graceful dance.

Tenesmus – A painfully urgent but ineffectual attempt to urinate or defecate.

Tonify – to strengthen or build.

Toxins – poisons; in Chinese Medicine this term often refers to the presence of bacteria or virus.

Ventilate (lungs) – to disperse energy stagnation in the lungs and to soothe breathing and help relieve cough and asthma.

Viscera – internal organs.

Warming food – one that reduces coldness in the body or is of a Yang nature; food that raises metabolism.

Wind – one of the external causes of disease; a syndrome characterized by fever, chills, head and body ache. Internal wind can disrupt the balance and manifest such symptoms as dizziness, fainting, convulsions, tremor, numbness, or pain that moves around (like the wind).

Wind cold – common cold or flu caused by the invasion of wind and cold. Symptoms are severe chills, mild fever, head and body ache, no sweat, and sinus congestion.

Wind heat – common cold or flu caused by the invasion of wind and heat. Symptoms are high fever, mild chills, sore throat, body and headache, sweating and thirst.

Yang – relating to the male, active, positive, fiery, energetic side of life or nature of a person.

Yang deficiency – a lack of heat or fire (Yang) within the body to counterbalance the water (Yin), characterized by coldness, Chi deficiency, tiredness, diarrhea with watery stools; a lack of energy to balance bodily substance.

Yin – relating to the female, passive, negative, watery, cool, substance side of life or nature of a person.

Yin deficiency – a lack of the coolness or water (Yin) within the body to counterbalance the fire (Yang), usually resulting in heat symptoms such as irritability, red cheeks, night sweats, dry cough, dry throat and insomnia; a lack of bodily substance to balance energy.

Bibliography

For further reading on the subjects of Traditional Chinese Medicine, Chinese nutrition, and the Taoist healing arts, we suggest the following books. Those books marked by an asterisk (*) supply additional information on Chinese herbs.

Traditional Chinese Medicine

*Beinfield, Harriet and Efrem Korngold. *Between Heaven and Earth: A Guide to Chinese Medicine.* New York: Random House Publishing (Ballantine Books), 1991.

Deng, Tietao. *Practical Diagnosis in Traditional Chinese Medicine.* Edinburgh: Churchill Livingstone, 2000.

Kaptchuk, Ted J. *The Web That Has No Weaver.* New York: McGraw-Hill, 2000.

L'Orange, Darlena with Gary Dolowich. *Ancient Roots, Many Branches.* Twin Lakes, WI: Lotus Press, 2002.

Maciocia, Giovanni. *The Foundations of Chinese Medicine,* Second Edition. New York: Elsevier (Churchill Livingstone), 2005.

Ni, Daoshing. *The Tao of Fertility.* New York: Collins (Harper-Colllins), 2008.

Ni, Maoshing. *Secrets of Self-Healing.* New York: Avery (Penguin Group), 2008.

Ni, Maoshing. *The Yellow Emperor's Classic of Medicine.* Boston and London: Shambhala, 1995.

*Unschuld, Paul. *Medicine in China: History of Pharmaceutics.* Berkeley, California: University of California Press, 1986.

Xinnong, Cheng. *Chinese Acupuncture and Moxibustion.* Bejing: Foreign Language Press, 1987.

Chinese Nutrition

Campbell, T. Colin and Thomas M. Campbell II, *The China Study.* Dallas, TX: BenBella Books, 2006.

Colbin, Annemarie. *Food and Healing.* New York: Ballantine Books, 1986.

Flaws, Bob and Honora Wolfe. *Prince Wen Hui's Cook: Chinese Dietary Therapy.* Brookline, Massachusetts: Paradigm Publications, 1983.

Haas, Elson. *Staying Healthy With the Seasons.* Berkeley, California: Celestial Arts, 2003.

Kastner, Joerg. *Chinese Nutrition Therapy: Dietetics in Traditional Chinese Medicine.* New York: Thieme, 2004.

Liu, Jilin and Gordon Peck. *Chinese Dietary Therapy.* London, England: Churchill Livingstone, 2004.

Lu, Henry C. *Chinese System of Food Cures.* New York: Sterling Publishing Co., 1986.

Lu, Henry C. *Chinese Natural Cures.* New York: Black Dog and Leventhal Publishers, 2005.

Pitchford, Paul. *Healing with Whole Foods: Asian Traditions and Modern Nutrition.* Berkeley, California: North Atlantic Books, 2002.

Zhang Enqin. *Chinese Medicated Diet.* Shanghai, China: Publishing House of Shanghai College of Traditional Chinese Medicine, 1988.

Chinese Herbs

Bensky, Dan, Steven Clavey, & Erich Stoger, *Chinese Herbal Medicine: Materia Medica, Third Edition*. Seattle: Eastland Press, 2004

Chen, John K. and Tina T. Chen. *Chinese Medical Herbology and Pharmacology*. City of Industry, CA: Art of Medicine Press, 2004.

Han, Henry, Glenn E. Miller, and Nancy Deville. *Ancient Herbs, Modern Medicine*. New York: Bantam Books, 2003.

Harrar, Sari and Sara Altshul O'Donnell. *Woman's Book of Healing Herbs*. Emmaus, PA: Rodale Press, 1999.

Hobbs, Christopher. *Medicinal Mushrooms*. Santa Cruz, CA: Botanica Press, 1995.

Holmes, Peter with Jing Wang. *The Traditional Chinese Medicine Materia Medica Clinical Reference and Study Guide*. Boulder, CO: Snow Lotus Press, 2002.

L'Orange, Darlena. *Herbal Healing Secrets of the Orient*. Paramus, NJ: Prentice Hall. 1998.

Ni, Maoshing. *Chinese Herbology Made Easy*. Los Angeles: SevenStar Communications, 1986.

Reid, Daniel. *A Handbook of Chinese Healing Herbs*. Boston, MA: Shambhala, 1995.

Teeguarden, Ron. *The Ancient Wisdom of the Chinese Tonic Herbs*. New York: Grand Central Publishing, 2000.

Tierra, Lesley. *Healing with Chinese Herbs*. Freedom, CA: The Crossing Press, 1997.

Tierra, Lesley. *Healing with the Herbs of Life*. Berkeley, CA: The Crossing Press, 2003.

Tierra, Michael. *The Way of Chinese Herbs*. New York: Pocket Books, 1998.

Tillotson, Alan Keith with Nai-shing Hu Tillotson and Robert Abel, Jr. *The One Earth Herbal Source Book: Everything You Need to Know about Chinese, Western, and Ayurvedic Herbal Treatments*. New York: Kensington Publishing, 2001.

Taoist Healing Arts

Jou, Tsung Hwa. *The Tao of T'ai Chi Ch'uan: Way to Rejuvenation*. Piscataway, New Jersey: T'ai Chi Foundation, 1983.

Liu, Da. *Taoist Health Exercises Book*. New York: Perigee Books, 1983.

Ming-dao, Deng. *Scholar Warrior: An Introduction to the Tao in Everyday Life*. San Francisco: HarperCollins, 1990.

Ni, Hua Ching. *8000 Years of Wisdom: Conversations With Taoist Master Ni*, Hua Ching, Vol. 1. Los Angeles: SevenStar Communications, 1995.

Ni, Hua Ching. *Tao, The Subtle Universal Law and Integral Way of Life*. Los Angeles: SevenStar Communications, 2003.

Ni, Maoshing. *Dr. Mao's Harmony Tai Chi*. San Francisco: Chronicle Books, 2006.

Ni, Maoshing. *Secrets of Longevity: Hundreds of Ways to Live to Be 100*. San Francisco: Chronicle Books, 2006.

Companion Cookbooks

The following book is a companion cookbook to The Tao of Nutrition *that utilizes the principles of Chinese nutrition and includes recipes with Chinese food herbs:*

Chuang, Lily. *Chinese Vegetarian Delights: Sugar and Dairy Free Cookbook.* Los Angeles: SevenStar Communications, 1987.

Chuang, Lily and Cathy McNease. *101 Vegetarian Delights.* Los Angeles: SevenStar Communications, 1992.

Cookbooks

Colbin, Annemarie. *The Book of Whole Meals.* New York: Ballantine Books, 1985.

Conrad, Kendall. *Eat Well Feel Well.* New York: Clarkson Potter, 2006.

Compestine, Ying Chang. *Secrets from a Healthy Asian Kitchen.* New York: Penguin Putnum, 2002.

Estella, Mary. *Natural Foods Cookbook: Vegetarian Dairy-Free Cuisine.* New York: Japan Publications, 1985.

Fessler, Stella Lau. *Chinese Meatless Cooking.* New York: Signet Books, 1983.

Flaws, Bob. *The Book of Jook.* Boulder, Colorado: Blue Poppy Press, 2007.

Haas, Elson M. *The New Detox Diet: The Complete Guide for Lifelong Vitality with Receipes, Menus, & Detox Plans.* Berkeley/Toronto: Celestial Arts, 2004.

Hagler, Louise. *Tofu Cookery.* Summertown, Tennessee: The Book Publishing Co., 2008.

Hou, FaXiang. *Unleashing the Power of Food: Recipes to Heal By.* Baltimore, Maryland: Agora Health Books, 2003.

Jacobs, Barbara and Leonard. *Cooking with Seitan: The Complete Vegetarian "Wheat-Meat" Cookbook.* New York: Avery, 1994.

Kafka, Barbara with Christopher Styler. *Vegetable Love.* New York: Workman Publishing, 2005.

Lappe, Frances Moore. *Diet for a Small Planet.* New York: Ballantine Books, 1991.

Leggett, Daverick. *Recipes for Self-Healing.* Totnes, England: Meridian Press, 1999

Lin, Florence. *Florence Lin's Chinese Vegetarian Cookbook.* Boulder, Colorado: Shambhala, 1983.

Madison, Deborah. *Vegetable Soups from Deborah Madison's Kitchen.* New York: Broadway Books, 2006.

Ody, Penelopy. *The Chinese Herbal Cookbook: Healing Foods for Inner Balance.* Trumbull, CT: Weatherhill, 2001.

Pickarski, Brother Ron. *Friendly Foods.* Berkeley, California: Ten Speed Press, 1991.

Robertson, Laurel, Carol Flinders, and Brian Ruppenthal. *The New Laurel's Kitchen.* Berkeley, California: Ten Speed Press, 1986.

Saltzman, Joanne. *Amazing Grains: Creating Vegetarian Main Dishes from Whole Grains.* Tiburon, California: H.J. Kramer, 1990.

Shurtleff, William and Akiko Aoyagi. *The Book of Tofu*. Berkeley, California: Ten Speed Press, 2001.

Turner, Lisa. *Meals That Heal.* Rochester, Vermont: Healing Arts Press, 1996.

Weber, Marcea. *Whole Meals.* Newberry Park, California: Prism Press, 1983.

Zhao, Zhuo and George Ellis. *The Healing Cuisine of China.* Rochester, VT: Healing Arts Press, 1998.

Sources for Chinese Food & Herbs

Some of the foods and herbs mentioned are only available from Asian markets, health food stores or specialty food stores. Chinatown in any large city will have the foods and herbs mentioned. Or, you may find sources by searching online for Chinese food or Chinese herbs. You can also look in the yellow pages of your local telephone directory. The following stores are potential sources for the Chinese foods and herbs recommended in this book:

www.asianfoodgrocer.com
www.99RanchMarket.com
(includes a directory of over 25 stores)

99 Ranch Market
6450 N. Sepulveda Blvd.
Van Nuys, CA 91411
(818) 988-7899

Wing Hop Fung
727 N. Broadway
Los Angeles, CA 90012
(213) 626-7200

99 Ranch Market
22511 Highway 99
Edmonds, WA 98026

Best Blends Herbs
PO Box 1329
Ojai, CA 93023
(805) 798-1107
Email: cathymcnease@hotmail.com

Tak Shing Hong
835 N. Broadway
Los Angeles, CA 90012
(213) 628-83333

Tin Bo Co.
841 N. Broadway
Los Angeles, CA 90012
(213) 680-3395

Traditions of Tao Herbal Supplements
13315 W. Washington Blvd., Ste. 200
Los Angeles, CA 90066
www.taostar.com

INDEX

Please note: A listing in boldface means the page contains a major heading. When Liver, Heart, Spleen, Lungs, and Kidneys are capitalized, they refer to the organ system in Chinese medicine.

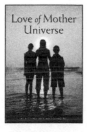

Love of Mother Universe—Imagine a life without artificial goodness, without fear and without social divisions. This work lays the foundation for a global society that honors the natural rhythms, subtle laws and sacred unity of the Mother Universe. It is from this universal perspective that you can make a real and lasting contribution to humanity.

304 pages. Available in softcover and digital formats.

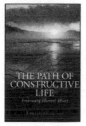

The Path of Constructive Life: Embracing Heaven's Heart—Unveils the new vehicle of the Integral Way known as The Path of Constructive Life. It gives fresh direction and effective self-practices to achieve sexual harmony, emotional well-being, protection from harmful influences and a universal soul.

315 pages. Available in softcover and digital formats.

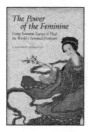

The Power of the Feminine: Using Feminine Energy to Heal the World's Spiritual Problems—The feminine approach is the true foundation of human civilization and spiritual growth. When positive feminine virtues are usurped in favor of masculine strength, aggression results. This book touches on how and why this imbalance occurs and encourages women to apply their gentle feminine virtue.

270 pages. Available in softcover and digital formats.

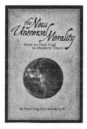

The New Universal Morality: How to Find God in Modern Times—An in-depth look at living in accord with universal virtue. Authors Hua-Ching Ni and Maoshing Ni, Ph.D. reveal a natural religion in which universal morality is the essence, the true God that supports our lives and all existence. Included is a discussion on the process of becoming a spiritual coach to serve both our community and ourselves.

280 pages. Available in softcover and digital formats.

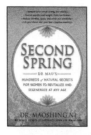

Second Spring: Dr. Mao's Hundreds of Natural Secrets For Women to Revitalize and Rejunvenate at Any Age—This tip-filled guide for women shows how to enhance energy, sexuality and health, especially during the second half of life. Dr. Maoshing Ni invites women to fulfill their innate potential and be at their most vital, energetic and attractive.

264 pages. Available in softcover and digital formats.

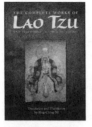

The Complete Works of Lao Tzu—The *Tao Teh Ching* is one of the most widely translated and cherished works of literature. Its timeless wisdom provides a bridge to the subtle spiritual truth and assists you to live harmoniously and peacefully. Also included is the *Hua Hu Ching*, a later work by Lao Tzu which has been lost to the general public for a thousand years.

212 pages. Available in softcover and digital formats.

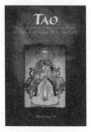

Tao, the Subtle Universal Law—Most people are unaware that their thoughts and behavior evoke responses from the invisible net of universal energy. To lead a good stable life is to be aware of the universal subtle law in every moment of our lives. This book presents practical methods that have been successfully used for centuries to accomplish this.

208 pages. Available in softcover and digital formats.

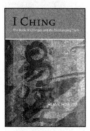

I Ching, The Book of Changes and the Unchanging Truth—This legendary classic is recognized as the first written book of wisdom. Leaders and sages throughout history have consulted it as a trusted advisor, which reveals the appropriate action in any circumstance. Includes over 200 pages of background material on natural energy cycles, instruction and commentaries.

669 pages, hardcover.

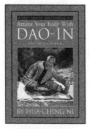

Attune Your Body with Dao-In—The ancients discovered that Dao-In exercises solved problems of stagnant energy, increased their health and lengthened their years. The exercises are also used as practical support for cultivation and higher achievements of spiritual immortality.

144 pages. Available in softcover and digital formats.

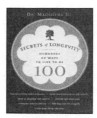

Secrets of Longevity: Hundreds of Ways To Live To Be 100— Looking to live a longer, happier, healthier life? Try eating more blueberries, telling the truth, and saying no to undue burdens. Dr. Maoshing Ni brings together simple and unusual ways to live longer.

320 pages. Available in softcover and digital formats.

Published by Chronicle Books

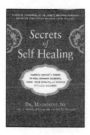

Secrets of Self-Healing—This landmark book on natural healing combines the wisdom of thousands of years of Eastern tradition with the best of modern medicine. Learn to treat common ailments with foods and herbs, and balance your mind and body to create vitality, wellness, and longevity.

576 pages. Available in softcover and digital formats.

Published by Penguin Group

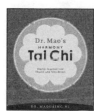

Dr. Mao's Harmony Tai Chi: Simple Practice for Health and Well-Being—This book focuses on awakening the spirit while strengthening the body. Ideal for both beginners and those looking to deepen their spiritual understanding of t'ai chi practice. Dr. Mao skillfully and clearly outlines the eighteen foundational movements.

124 pages. Published by Chronicle Books

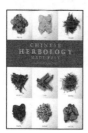

Chinese Herbology Made Easy—This text provides an overview of Oriental Medical theory, in-depth descriptions of each herb category, over 300 black and white photographs, extensive tables of individual herbs for easy reference and an index of pharmaceutical names.

202 pages, softcover.

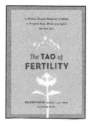

The Tao of Fertility: A Healing Chinese Medicine Program to Prepare Body, Mind, and Spirit for New Life—Dr. Daoshing Ni, an esteemed doctor who has helped countless women achieve their dream of having a child, offers his program for enhancing fertility through Traditional Chinese Medicine (TCM) and Taoist principles.

304 pages, softcover. Published by Collins

To order: 800-772-0222 ❧ www.taostar.com

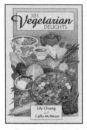

101 Vegetarian Delights—by Lily Chuang and Cathy McNease. From exotic flavorful feast to nutritious everyday meal, enjoy preparing these easy-to-make recipes. Based on the ancient Chinese tradition of balance and harmony, these dishes were created for the new or seasoned vegetarian. The desserts are truly delightful, and healthy as well.

176 pages, softcover.

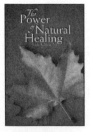

Power of Natural Healing—Hua-Ching Ni discusses the natural capability of self-healing and presents methods of cultivation–practices that can assist any treatment method–which promote a healthy life, longevity, and spiritual achievement. There is a natural healing process inherent in the very nature of life itself. One's own spirit is the source of health.

143 pages. Available in softcover and digital formats.

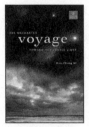

The Uncharted Voyage Toward the Subtle Light—This book provides a profound understanding and insight into the underlying heart of all paths of spiritual growth, the subtle origin, and the eternal truth of one universal life. Readers will enter a voyage of discovery, finding a fresh new light toward which to direct their life energy.

424 pages. Available in softcover and digital formats.

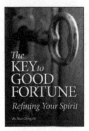

The Key to Good Fortune: Refining Your Spirit (Revised)—"Straighten your Way" (*Tai Shan Kan Yin Pien*) and "The Silent Way of Blessing" (*Yin Chi Wen*) are the main guidance for a mature, healthy life. Spiritual improvement can be an integral part of realizing a Heavenly life on earth.

153 pages. Available in softcover and digital formats.

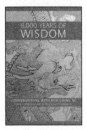

8,000 Years of Wisdom, Volume I and II
This two-volume set contains a wealth of practical, down-to-earth advice given by Hua-Ching Ni. Drawing on his training in Traditional Chinese Medicine, herbology and acupuncture, Hua-Ching Ni gives candid answers to questions on many topics.
Vol. I: (Revised edition) Includes dietary guidance.
Vol. II: Sex and pregnancy guidance.

Resources

College of Tao & Integral Health
Distance Learning Courses

Traditional Chinese Medicine: Concepts of Chinese Nutrition
Includes DVD and course materials
CEU credit available
800-772-0222
taostar@taostar.com

Achieve a basic understanding of Chinese nutrition theories and its practical applications. In four illustrated manuals, topics covered are food energetics, Zang-Fu syndromes, diagnosis and nutrition counseling, food choices for specific illnesses, and patient education. Please contact us for a brochure.

Traditional Chinese Medicine (TCM) Studies
Includes audio CD and all self-study materials
800-772-0222
taostar@taostar.com
www.collegeoftao.org

Listen to lectures by exceptional instructors. Each course includes notes for home study and appropriate reading and/or journal assignments, charts, textbooks, or herb samples. For personal interest; not a certificate program. Courses include:

Chinese Herbology
Traditional Chinese Medicine Theory: I, II, III
Chinese Acupuncture Points
Becoming a TCM Healer
The Power of Natural Healing

Please contact us for updates and a brochure.

Spiritual Self-Development: The Integral Way of Life
Internet study
info@taostudies.com
www.taostar.com

People who have read one or more books on the Integral Way of Life will find support in this study program. Having deepened their understanding and experience of the Way, students will learn how to live a constructive path of life.

Yo San University of Traditional Chinese Medicine

13315 W. Washington Boulevard, 2nd floor
Los Angeles, CA 90066
877-967-2648; 310-577-3000
www.yosan.edu

One of the finest and most academically rigorous Traditional Chinese Medical schools in the United States, Yo San University offers a fully accredited Master's degree program in acupuncture, herbology, *tui na* body work, and *chi* movement arts. In this program, students explore their spiritual growth as an integral part of learning the healing arts.

Tao of Wellness, Inc.

310-917-2200
www.taoofwellness.com

The Tao of Wellness center for Traditional Chinese Medicine is the integral way to total well-being and a long life. Each patient is seen as an individual whose health is immediately affected by his or her lifestyle including diet, habits, emotions, attitude, and environment. The center, co-founded by Drs. Daoshing and Maoshing Ni, focuses on acupuncture and Chinese herbs for complete health, longevity, and fertility.

Chi Health Institute

PO Box 2035
Santa Monica, California 90406-2035
www.taostar.com

The Chi Health Institute (CHI) offers professional education and certification in the Ni family *chi* movement arts including *tai chi, chi gong,* and Taoist meditation.

Integral Way Society

PO Box 1530
Santa Monica, CA 90406-1530
www.taostar.com

Learn about natural spiritual teachings as transmitted by the Ni family through books, mentoring, and retreats organized by the mentors of the Integral Way. The IWS assists people in achieving physical, mental, spiritual, moral and financial health by nurturing self-respect and by offering methods of self-improvement based on the principles in the classic works of the *I Ching* and Lao Tzu's *Tao Teh Ching.*

InfiniChi Institute International

PO Box 26712
San Jose, CA 95159-6712
408-295-5911
www.taostar.com

Professional training in *chi* healing leads to certification as an InfiniChi practitioner. The program is designed to develop your energetic healing abilities utilizing the Ni family books and texts that relate to Traditional Chinese Medicine, *chi gong,* Chinese bodywork, and natural spirituality. It features a progressive, systematic program that nurtures understanding, facilitates skill development, and promotes self-growth.

Acupuncture.com

www.acupuncture.com

Acupuncture.com is the gateway to Chinese medicine, health, and wellness. From this site you can purchase Tao of Wellness herbal products, choose from a large selection of traditional formulas and buy acupuncture books and related products.